Shattered to Strong

A SHIFT IN **TBI RECOVERY** ROOTED IN SCIENCE

SHATTERED TO STRONG

A SHIFT IN **TBI RECOVERY** ROOTED IN SCIENCE

PHYSICS, PHYSIOLOGY,
AND SELF-EXPERIENCE

"WHY MY TRAUMATIC BRAIN INJURY
WAS THE BEST THING TO EVER HAPPEN TO ME"

JOSEPH DITURI, PhD, CDR, U.S.
NAVY SATURATION DIVER (RET)

VIKING STONE PRESS

Shattered to Strong: A Shift in TBI Recovery Rooted in Science
Published by Viking Stone Press
Tampa, Florida, U.S.A.

Disclaimer:
This book has not been cleared for open production, and the views expressed in this publication are the author's own and do not necessarily reflect the official position of the Department of Defense or the United States government, nor the University of South Florida or any other organization with which the author may be affiliated. It is a no-nonsense, unbiased personal look at an innovative way to heal traumatic brain injury.

The information contained in this book is not medical advice. Dr. Joseph Dituri is not a Medical Doctor or Doctor of Osteopathic Medicine. The reader is advised to seek advice from a medical doctor before attempting any treatments referenced in this book.

Library of Congress Control Number: 2026915098

DITURI, JOSEPH, Author
SHATTERED TO STRONG
JOSEPH DITURI, Ph.D., CDR, US Navy (Ret)

ISBN: 979-8-9853664-4-0 (paperback)
ISBN: 979-8-9853664-5-7 (digital)

BIOGRAPHY & AUTOBIOGRAPHY / Doctors
HEALTH & FITNESS / Diseases & Conditions / Brain
TECHNOLOGY & ENGINEERING / Biomedical

Cover Image: Brian P. O'Connell, EdD, CW4 U.S. Army (Ret)
Editing: Bethany Good, (goodwritingco.com)
Book Design & E-book formatting: Amit Dey (amitdey2528@gmail.com)
Project Management & Consulting: Susie Schaefer (finishthebookpublishing.com)

DEDICATION

To Rear Admiral Edward Winters, United States Navy
(SEAL) (Ret)
June 1956 – June 2026

Dear Ed,

Your wisdom, strength, and quiet guidance
shaped me more than you ever knew.

This book exists because of the foundation
you helped me build.

Thank you, my friend.
Fair winds and following seas.

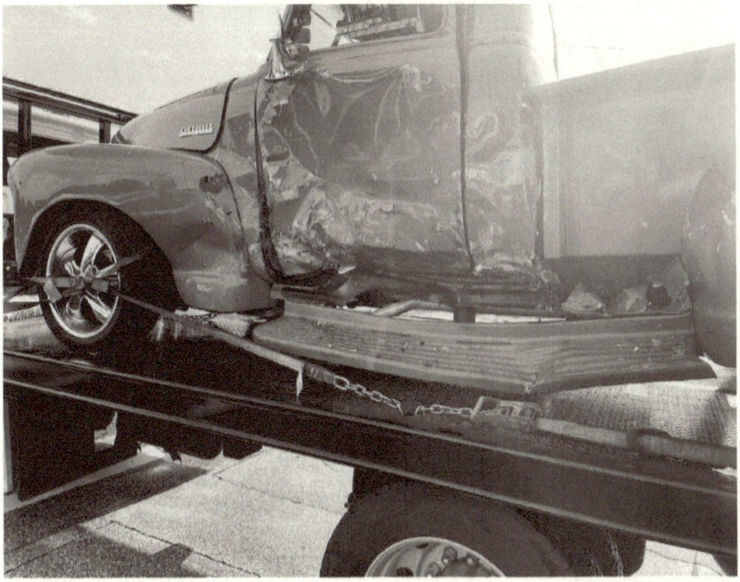

TABLE OF CONTENTS

A NOTE FROM THE AUTHOR

I want to share a little bit about myself. After 28 years of active service to the United States, I earned a PhD in Biomedical Engineering with research areas of interest that include life support equipment design, high carbon dioxide environments, as well as hyperbaric and hypobaric medicine. My areas of interest are broad and include studying undersea environments and ocean conservation. This book will focus on traumatic brain injury (TBI) and the treatments I have tested on myself. I am dedicated to understanding TBI and helping sufferers and the people that care for them understand this injury better. I am a professor of medical engineering at the University of South Florida with a vested interest in Veterans Health Research. My research areas are Traumatic Brain Injury and Healthspan. My lab is a Center of Excellence for Research into Anti-Aging, Brain Repair, Hyperbaric and Hypobaric Medicine.

I'd like to introduce a no-nonsense approach to writing this book. At the beginning of every chapter, I intend to put the following four letters: BLUF. That is an acronym for Bottom Line Up Front (BLUF). It's a powerful briefing tool I learned in the military. Leaders want a no-nonsense overview prior to getting into the details. This helps keep the "end in mind," a sentiment popularized by William Edwards Deming, an American industrial engineer, management consultant, statistician, and Ph.D.

He is also known as the father of the quality movement. He is best known for his theories of management. The thought is that if you understand where the chapter is going (Quo Vadis in Latin), you can gain a better conceptualization of the complex topic at hand.

INTRODUCTION

The best thing in disguise…and why my TBI was the best thing that ever happened.

BLUF – My TBI gave me a new way of looking at an age-old problem with hope for a path to resolution. The hope herein is that the reader will embrace a new methodology for working with those who suffer from TBI.

Can a traumatic brain injury be the best thing to ever happen to someone? The answer is a resounding YES. My traumatic brain injury (TBI) became the catalyst for transforming my mind, body, and spirit. This book explores how a TBI can lead not only to a better, more meaningful life, but also answers that can provide hope and healing for others still suffering from this literal pandemic.

The brain, an incredible organ located within the skull, is a tangible part of the body made up of neurons, glial cells, and other tissues. It serves as the biological hardware that controls bodily functions, processes sensory input, and supports cognitive processes. The mind, however, is an abstract concept, referring to the collection of processes and activities, such as thoughts, consciousness, emotions, perceptions, and memories, that arise from the brain's activity. While the brain is the physical structure enabling these functions, the mind is the subjective experience and output of the neural processes. For example, the brain's neural firing patterns can be measured using tools like the electroencephalogram (EEG), which can reveal phenomena such as decision-making and self-awareness. However, outside of measuring brain activity, self-awareness and the like are not directly observable. The distinction between the brain and the mind lies in the brain being the material substrate and the mind being the functional or experiential result. Their exact relationship remains a topic of debate in neuroscience and philosophy.

TBI has been recognized as a medical issue in scientific literature for centuries. Ancient medical texts, such as the Edwin Smith Papyrus (around 1700 BC), describe head injuries and their symptoms, indicating early awareness of TBI's effects.[1] The term "concussion" was used in medical contexts as early as the 16th century. But systematic research into TBI as a distinct condition did not accelerate until the early 20th century, particularly during World War I, when "shell shock" cases prompted studies on brain trauma from blast injuries.[2] By the 1980s, advancements in neuroimaging (e.g., CT scans) and standardized classifications like the Glasgow Coma Scale (1974) had solidified TBI as a major focus in neuroscience and medicine. With this also came growing recognition of its long-term effects, such as chronic traumatic encephalopathy (CTE), which was notably studied in the 2000s. TBI has been referenced as a problem for millennia… that's right, for thousands of years. Rigorous scientific study spans roughly the last 150 years, with only minimal progress in the past 50 years. We can do better!

[1] Burridge. (July 2007)

[2] Lindberg. (August 25, 2022)

TBI sufferers may experience a persistent "fight or flight" response due to neurological and psychological changes caused by the injury. I certainly did. TBIs often affect brain regions, such as the amygdala and prefrontal cortex, that regulate emotions and stress responses. Damage can lead to an overactive amygdala, triggering heightened alertness or hyperarousal, a hallmark of the fight-or-flight response. This is demonstrated by an increase in amygdala size and a decrease in hippocampal volume.

I had a 28-year career in the Navy and have worked with many veterans during my time researching TBI. Veterans with TBI are also more likely to have post-traumatic stress disorder (PTSD), which amplifies fight-or-flight responses. The combination of TBI and PTSD can make it difficult to "turn off" the stress response, as traumatic memories or triggers keep the brain in survival mode. TBI can impair cognitive processing and sensory filtering, making every day stimuli feel overwhelming. This can cause the brain to misinterpret neutral situations as threats, activating the fight-or-flight response. Finally, military training and combat experiences condition veterans to stay vigilant. TBI can exacerbate this, making it hard for the brain to adapt to non-threatening civilian environments, leaving veterans stuck in a stress response loop. Overall, they are dealing with a highly fictional but seemingly factual occurrence. That recursive loop must be stopped, or the sufferer must be taught to control it.

Most military people think differently compared with the rest of the population. The well-being and freedom of one's compadres or friends is often a more immediate and concrete motivator than abstract notions of national freedom. This perspective leads to stronger bonds and more effective cohesive action during difficult or stressful times, such as battle. This idea is akin to the concept of "buddy care" or the importance of unit cohesion. Military members are often more motivated to fight for their friends and comrades than for a cause they may not fully understand or believe in. Overall, this is a call to prioritize the human element in warfare and to recognize that the freedom of the individual soldier is intrinsically linked to the freedom of the group. However, the human element is completely ignored when we treat former military members with TBI. When we diagnose or treat veterans and service members for TBI, we often fail to consider their unique psychology, which can have disastrous results.

Presently, there is no cure for TBI. The U.S. Food and Drug Administration (FDA) has not approved any pharmacological or device-based treatment that can fully reverse or cure TBI.[3] The concept of a "cure" for TBI is complex, given the range of outcomes from mild to severe cases. Even in mild cases, there is the possibility of persistent symptoms or later neurodegenerative risks. The best we can do after fighting this for thousands of years is:

- Symptom reduction or alleviation
- Functional improvement
- Preventing a secondary injury

While the scientific method is important, I believe we need a better model to research TBI. Using the scientific method of only changing one variable when testing does not allow us to fully understand the complex nature of TBI. These drug companies can easily isolate a proposed treatment, giving a red pill

[3] FDA. "Traumatic Brain Injury: What to Know About Symptoms, Diagnosis, and Treatment"

or blue pill, completely making it easy for them, and them alone. I don't want to throw all the science out the window, but the limitations of only focusing on one variable is a critical consideration. The problem has become systemic, and it keeps getting worse. We need to have a watershed moment when it comes to doing research; we need to look at how to move the needle to help somebody. The scientific community is just going to need to get on board with accepting the fact that they have had thousands of years to repair this and have come up with absolutely nothing. That's right, despite millennia of trying to find a cure, we still have none.

What the medical community has been doing until now is not working. We need something better. We may never find the best way to solve this issue, but we need to know which treatment modalities are most effective. Unquestionably, we need to make changes to the way that we've been doing things. We need to know which treatment modalities are most effective. However, we need to make changes to the way that we've been doing things. I teach a course at medical school and have great insight into human physiology. I believe the way that we have been doing it simply does not work, and that means we need to do it differently.

As a clinical researcher and someone who has reviewed, discussed, and evaluated thousands of TBIs, I assure you that each and every one of them differs vastly. It is and always has been my affirmation that "*if you have seen one TBI ... you have seen one TBI.*" This is a fact. I believe in and have experienced great success with a simultaneously applied multi-therapeutic approach. Though your path to recovery is significantly different from my path, I feel a common truth in the methods of healing. I started with these simple premises:

- Do no harm to myself
- Increase cerebral blood flow
- Science wins over bullshit
- If we had the fix, we would have solved this by now
- What works…. works
- Multiple therapies simultaneously applied have a greater impact than a single therapy

It is apparent to me that anyone with a TBI needs to grab the bull by the horns and prioritize self-care. It is important for the reader to understand that whatever they have been doing up until now is not working, so they should do *something* … *anything* different. Start by changing the people you spend time with and prioritize surrounding yourself with positive people. Go to the gym or go for a walk… go do *something*. Find some purpose and save yourself. Importantly, the overriding answer to this question posed at the head of this introduction is "YES… your TBI can be the best thing that's ever happened to you." It takes some good, hard looking at yourself, answering some really difficult questions, and changing the way you think. As Buddha says, "The mind is everything. What you think, you become."

This book is my narrative: an educated medical and systematic approach to treating TBI, shaped by my journey as both a researcher and a patient. It's a roadmap for surviving the unimaginable, for finding a way forward after being stripped bare by injury or illness, and for rebuilding a life of purpose and hope.

CHAPTER ONE

When the Light Turned Green

"Unspoken expectations are premeditated resentment."

- Anne Lamott, Author

BLUF – My life changed the moment the traffic light turned green, and I had to learn to live with the changes. The Creator decided to wake me up by knocking me out.

I pressed the accelerator, ready to move forward, but The Creator had other plans. A 6,000-pound SUV barreled into me at full speed, t-boning my truck at a busy Tampa intersection on September 7th of 2021. In an instant, everything I thought I knew about life, medicine, and myself came to a screeching halt.

After 28 years in the U.S. Navy, specializing in hyperbaric medicine, and nearly a decade studying and teaching biomedical engineering, I believed I had the answers. I thought I knew how to treat TBI. For years, I had devoted my career to helping military members who were either slowly dying from PTSD and TBI or ending their suffering quickly with a bullet to the brain. But I did not have all the answers—not yet.

When I regained consciousness, I was no longer Professor Joseph Dituri. I was not the expert, the healer, or the man with solutions. I was the patient. I was the one lying in a hospital bed with a brain bleed and a TBI of my own. The roles had reversed, and I was not ready. Traditional medicine did not work for me. It was not enough for the damage I had sustained. So, The Creator forced my hand. I had to save my own life.

Before the accident, I was focused. I was almost too focused. My sights were locked on curing TBI, and I was marching forward with conviction. It was a noble goal, but I see now that it was not enough. I was missing something fundamental: empathy. I thought I understood what my subjects were going through; however, in reality… I couldn't fully grasp their struggles.

The Good Lord had been whispering to me all along, nudging me toward a deeper understanding. "Joe, you need something more," he said, but I did not listen. I was stubborn. "No," I told myself. "I've got this…. What I'm doing is enough." When I ignored the whispers, God sent me a wake-up call with a message that could not be ignored.

"Joe," He said, "I asked you to do this when you were whole. Now, you'll have to do it while you're broken. You'll have to learn what it means to struggle, to suffer, and to fight your way back. Only then will you have the compassion and empathy to truly help others."

The accident wasn't just a tragedy; it was a transformation. It stripped me of my certainties, my pride, and my assumptions. But in doing so, it gave me something far greater: the chance to rebuild myself into someone who could not only heal but also truly understand.

It was 9:00 a.m., and I had just come back from the gym, feeling energized after my workout. I stopped by to chat with my mechanic about a loose spark plug that was making an odd noise in my 1947 Chevy pickup truck. I remember pulling up to a red light on Westshore Boulevard and coming to a stop.

All I recall is that several moments later, the light turned green and I hit the gas. And then… nothing. I do not remember the truck that slammed into me or the collision itself. The details are a black hole in my memory, swallowed by the impact.

My truck, a 1947 Chevy with shaved door handles and pop locks, had a major design flaw in moments like this: the doors couldn't be opened from the outside. When the first responders arrived, I was dazed, unable to unlock the doors myself. A brave bystander, whom I met later, stepped in to help the firefighter rip the door open.

This same man, a fellow car enthusiast, quickly recognized an even greater danger. My truck's engine had stalled in the crash, but the ignition key was still turned on, powering the electronic fuel pump. Gasoline continued flooding into the hot, damaged carburetor, creating a serious fire hazard that could have put the entire intersection at risk. Thankfully, this Good Samaritan acted fast and cut the fuel pump before disaster struck.

I learned of this man's heroism much later. At a TBI charity event, a stranger approached me and asked, "Were you recently in a bad accident?" He then asked me how I was recovering, and recounted the entire story, mourning the loss of my beautiful truck. Before I could properly thank him, he slipped away into the crowd. I never caught his name. He's now just another fragment in the sea of memories that have slipped through the cracks of time.

Back to the morning of the accident… At some point during the chaos I regained consciousness, but I could immediately tell my mind was not working how it did before the accident. The details of what happened were jumbled and incomplete. I remember that my administrative assistant, who worked just three blocks away, came running to the scene.

She knelt beside me, saying, "Oh my God, are you ok?"

I looked at her blankly. "Do I know you?" I asked. She was heartbroken because I did not even recognize her.

I was transported by ambulance to St. Joseph's Hospital in Tampa. The ride itself is a blur. I'm told I called a few people during the trip, insisting I was fine. "What happened?" they asked. "Nothing happened," I said.

When we arrived at the hospital, a young neurosurgeon walked into the room and greeted me with, "Hey, Doc." He looked like he was twelve years old. It turned out he had been one of my students at some point, but I couldn't quite place him. He explained my condition in clinical terms: an eight-millimeter hemorrhagic stroke in the prefrontal cortex.

"We may need to drill a hole in your head," he said casually. That sounded like a terrible idea, and I didn't hesitate to tell him so. He decided to observe me in the ICU instead.

Those two days in the ICU were some of the longest of my life. I was labeled a fall risk, confined to bed, and unable to do anything without assistance. As a former special operations diving officer, I was used to solving problems and taking charge, but now, I could not even go to the bathroom without someone holding my hand. It was a humbling experience.

And yet, when I pushed the call button for assistance, no one came. After waiting too long, I decided to get up on my own. The bed sensors betrayed me. Alarms blared, and within seconds, two nurses came running in. They scolded me like a child, lecturing me on why I needed to wait for help. The staff seemed to move at a speed just faster than glacial. I nodded along, but inside, I was screaming. How did it come to this? How had I gone from being the person everyone relied on to someone who couldn't even rely on himself?

After two days in the ICU, the neurosurgeon informed me that my intracranial pressure had stabilized, meaning at least it hadn't worsened. That was enough for me to be downgraded to a regular hospital room. While this felt like a step forward, I was still on fall-risk status. At least by this point, I was able to use the restroom alone, albeit with an escort required for the walk. Small victories, I thought.

I spent another five or six days in the hospital, the entire time begging to be discharged. Slowly, the fog of my memory began to lift, and I realized the young neurosurgeon was not just someone I had taught; he had been a friend. By the time I left the hospital, that realization had settled in, but my sense of identity had not.

When I was finally released on September 14th of 2021, it came with strict orders: go home, go to bed, and do nothing else. But I had my other plans. I was determined to fix my brain using the same methods I'd been advocating for years to help TBI victims.

I set off on my same old path, determined to follow the protocols I'd spent years developing. Deep down, though, I knew this approach wouldn't be enough. It wasn't that the methods didn't work; they did, but they weren't tailored for someone like me, someone broken in ways I couldn't yet comprehend. Still, I stuck to my routine. I clung to the familiar even though it wasn't serving me. It would take months, and more than a few dark nights contemplating ending it all, before I finally stepped off that road and onto a new one.

To better understand why we need to approach brain injuries differently, think of a hidden plumbing leak as an analogy. When a small water stain appears on a ceiling, you have some idea that a water leak exists somewhere inside. However, even with sophisticated moisture sensors, the true source of a pinhole leak in a specific pipe remains invisible until a plumber opens the wall to find the problem. The brain, however, is infinitely more complex than a water leak behind your wall, and opening a person's skull is rarely an option. This forces us to rely on limited external views from MRIs or CT scans, even as hidden internal processes continue to cause problems.

Neurosurgeons and neurologists do not "get inside" your brain unless it is a life-or-death emergency. This makes imaging, our best non-invasive diagnostic tool, critically important but inherently limited. Despite the brain's complexities, we remain reliant on tools that provide only a snapshot in time, and lack the dynamic, temporal data needed to reveal critical details such as blood flow and neural connectivity.

The inability to fully visualize or comprehend the intricacies of the brain shouldn't prevent us from exploring innovative treatments. By acknowledging the limitations of current imaging technologies and being willing to embrace alternative measures, including subjective observations such as electroencephalogram (EEG), we could open new doors for TBI, PTSD, and other neurological conditions.

Unfortunately, hubris often stands in the way of such advancements. Many in the medical field hesitate to admit that our understanding of the brain is incomplete. Yet, the reality is clear: imaging alone cannot provide the full picture of what is happening inside the brain. Just as knee surgeons approach surgery with the understanding that they will not know the full extent of the problem until they're inside, neurologists and neurosurgeons must accept that they, too, are operating with an incomplete view.

This lack of clarity demands a broader, more flexible approach to evidence, one that incorporates both objective and subjective measures. Until we develop technologies that allow us to "get in there" non-invasively and in real time, we must lean on every tool and observation available to us, even if it challenges traditional medical protocols.

Instead of asking, "How do we cure TBI?" we can reframe the question to something far more impactful: "How can we help the patient?" By listening to the patient's story, we can begin to understand not just the medical challenges they face but the social, emotional, and psychological hurdles as well. This holistic approach shifts the focus to treating the whole person, using methods that are often unconventional in traditional medicine.

Adopting this mindset requires a leap of faith, a willingness to challenge the prevailing notion that time is the only "cure" for a traumatic brain injury. When I was first diagnosed, a practitioner told me exactly that: "The only cure is the tincture of time." The dismissal in those words enraged me. As a sailor, I was trained to "spit" (metaphorically) in the face of adversity or danger, and this was no different. Time alone was not going to fix me.

The truth is, medical providers often know very little about the individual who walks into their office. They do their best in the brief window they have, filling out forms, checking boxes, but a 10-minute visit is hardly enough to understand a person's life or challenges. The patient and their family, however, know the full story. They see the progress (or lack of it) every day. They often know best what works and what does not.

To illustrate this point, consider a potted plant. If you ask three people what is wrong with a wilting plant, one might say, "It needs water." Another might say, "It needs sunlight." A third could argue, "It needs fertilizer." In medical research, the current system often forces us to isolate confounding variables. We strip the plant of water and food, expose it to 24 hours of sunlight, and find it dies. The conclusion? Sunlight kills plants. Next, we remove sunlight and food, and the plant dies when exposed to only water. Again, we conclude water is harmful. Finally, we do the same with food and arrive at yet another flawed conclusion.

The problem with pharmaceutical-funded research is that it reduces the human experience to isolated variables and misses the bigger picture. In doing so, it fails to treat the whole person. Such research is so focused on dissecting the parts that it forgets to nurture the system as a whole. Humans intuitively know or understand that a combination of sunlight, water, and food is required for the overall health of a plant, and one is not necessarily more important than the other. As of early 2026, there are over 7,000[4] pharmaceutical companies worldwide with active research and development pipelines, with thousands of drugs in the global pipeline. That is likely the lion's share of all research accomplished and is most assuredly the issue at hand!

If we truly want to heal people, especially those with TBI, we need to abandon this fragmented approach and embrace

[4] A. Minhas. (May 11, 2026).

one that acknowledges the complexity of human beings. Listening to the patient's story and working with them as a partner in their care might not fit neatly into a study or satisfy a pharmaceutical model, but it's often the key to real healing.

While I was trying to fix my brain during a TBI, I was literally flying by the seat of my pants. I had to feel my way through repairing my own brain as though I were groping around in the dark. I had to set aside my emotions and retrain my clinical researcher mindset to find answers in physics and physiology. This was much like flying an airplane while assembling it. Logic and present medical standards of care have failed our society and me, and I needed to do something. I was completely despondent.

I realized that I needed to approach my TBI treatment on three different fronts: healing my physical body, as well as addressing my physiologic concerns and psychological concerns. Much like the plant analogy above, everything must be in balance; the only way to cure it is to treat all three simultaneously. If you only treat the patient psychologically, they still have remnants in their physical and physiologic parts, which continue to remind the brain they have a TBI. Without treating all these issues simultaneously and in the right amounts, healing isn't possible.

The current standard of care for traumatic brain injury is to diagnose and discharge. Why? The issue here is that magnetic resonance imaging (MRI), even with diffuse tensor imaging (MRI-DTI), only provides a momentary snapshot and does not represent the full or prolonged picture of what is happening in the brain.

After my accident, I tried to continue living normally while performing treatments on myself. These were treatments I had used on many others for years. One such method was hyperbaric oxygen therapy (HBOT), which I used for a month and a half following the incident. That method alone didn't work for me. By the end of October, I was in a downward spiral and in such a poor state that I was contemplating suicide. I felt there was no way out and became furious with myself. My emotional state worsened, and I found myself prone to uncontrollable crying.

I would sit alone in my office, isolated, as few people wanted to be around me by that point.

After 28 years of Naval service and the years I'd spent earning my Ph.D., I found myself unable to think my way out of the situation. I could not find a way through science, which left me feeling like an absolute failure.

One day, I was sitting in my office, overcome with tears, when my friend Travis paid me a visit. He immediately noticed I was in bad shape and, in an act of concern, called a psychiatrist he knew. My struggle to sleep had been compounding everything. Sleep deprivation is a common hallmark of TBIs. When the brain feels like it's not functioning properly, it refuses to shut off. Yet sleep is crucial for recovery and learning. The psychiatrist suggested medication to help me rest, a decision that… in hindsight… was pivotal. That much-needed, albeit drug-induced, sleep gave me the strength to begin seeking alternative forms of care.

Still fiercely holding onto my need for control, I resolved that if I were to end my life, I would first exhaust every avenue of healing I could find. I set a timeline for myself: by my birthday, December 8th, just over a month away, I would make my final decision. But first, I would apply every bit of knowledge I'd accumulated over my 28 years in the Navy and my academic career at the University of South Florida. I owed myself and my children that much before doing the unthinkable. Much later, this became my first critical learning point. Despair can come rapidly for those suffering from TBI.

A green light stopped me. But it has been a go ever since. My new platform and program allow me to offer the following advice to anyone with a friend or family member facing a TBI, PTSD, or other life-altering injury. Supporting someone through this journey can be challenging, but your understanding and compassion are critical.

How to support a loved one with a TBI:

1. **Empathize with them.** Understand that their behavior is often shaped by a dysregulation of brain pathways. They are not the same person they were before. Long-term memories you expect them to have may no longer be intact, and shared experiences may not be readily accessible to them. Patience and recognition go a long way. Keep in mind that many individuals with TBIs or PTSD hold onto a residual self-image. They are likely beating themselves up for not being as capable or well as they once were.
2. **Acknowledge intrusive thoughts.** TBI sufferers often experience intrusive, repetitive thoughts that they struggle to push away. Resistance can create a cyclical pattern, making the thoughts even more persistent. Help them work on acceptance rather than resisting or dismissing the thoughts. Avoid reassurances like, "Do not worry, this will get better." Instead, let them sit with the discomfort and gradually learn to coexist with

these thoughts. Regular check-ins can help ensure they do not dwell or spiral.

3. **Set boundaries for irrational or risk-taking behavior.** While empathy is essential, so is accountability. It's important to confront them with honesty and have frank discussions about their well-being. Make it clear that you want to help, but also set limits to protect them and others from harm.
4. **Treat each day as a global reset.** Do not assume they will remember what happened yesterday. Be patient, kind, and supportive, and prepare yourself to repeat things as often as necessary. Recovery is not linear, and walking beside them on this road takes resilience.
5. **Stay open to treatment options.** Explore every available method and remain hopeful. Innovation and unconventional therapies may provide breakthroughs. Do not lose faith in their ability to recover or adapt.

Finally, remember this: what may seem like the end is often just the beginning of a bolder and brighter future.

CHAPTER TWO

**Our future is anchored in our past.
From childhood to a "Life of Waivers".**

"There is nothing noble in being superior to your fellow man; true nobility is being superior to your former self."

-Ernest Hemingway

BLUF – This chapter explores the experiences that shaped my perspective as a university assistant professor and retired naval officer. I will tell you about my journey from a modest childhood through my time in the Navy and beyond. I will explain how I came to the belief that rules can be navigated creatively to achieve meaningful outcomes. This mindset, born of necessity, has guided me through personal and professional obstacles, including moments of self-doubt in the face of criticism.

I was born in Oceanside, New York, in December 1967. My early years were spent in Torino, Italy, where my father's job took our family. My father worked for an Italian company called Olivetti, where he converted documents from Italian to English. We returned to the United States in the early 1970s, settling in a modest home in Lindenhurst, Long Island, at the corner of 5th Street and 2nd Avenue. Money was tight, and school shopping meant one pair of jeans and a few shirts. This was in stark contrast to my more affluent high school peers. As the youngest of three boys, born within a year of each other, I grew up in a lively but resource-scarce household. A banner day was when my father installed a ventilation fan to combat New York's sweltering summers, as air conditioning was beyond our means.

Despite a largely happy childhood, I faced challenges. I had strabismus, commonly known as lazy eye, which led to frequent bullying. This lazy eye will become important again with my TBI. When I was in the sixth grade, my parents decided it was time to have surgery to correct this issue. I was getting into too many fights with bullies who smacked me and said, "Look at me when I am talking to you." Reminder: this was the dog-eat-dog world of public schools on Long Island, New York, in the 1970s. Some of these bullies were so good at their chosen profession that I would walk on the other side of the street or hall just to avoid them. They would take almost any opportunity to punch, kick, slap, or belittle anyone and everyone who was not in the cool kid's club, and my lazy eye and smaller stature had me planted firmly in the "not cool" club.

My parents' hope was that the surgery would correct my lazy eye and reduce the number of calls to the principal's office. For the most part, it did correct that lazy eye, but it also left me with a brief bout of double vision. Double vision is a normal occurrence from that lazy eye surgery, and it often corrects itself.

Throughout my childhood, I did not excel at school. Consequently, I basically loathed all things that were school-related, such as homework, reading, and so forth. I found reading very difficult. For instance, when I took the standardized aptitude test (SAT), I scored a whopping 910 out of a possible 1600 points. This prompted a guidance counselor to predict slim chances of my getting into college. I applied to several colleges and even got dressed in a suit for interviews, but I received only rejections, leaving me with zero college options.

I needed to figure out what I was going to do with my future. My friend, Brian O'Connell, and I would stand on the corner of 6th Street and 2nd Avenue hanging out and dreaming about "getting out" of that neighborhood. I could not stay on Long Island because it just wasn't for me, and I definitely did not want to get a job at my father's business, an audiovisual corporation. So, there wasn't anything left for me but a career in the military. I hate to use the term "forced," but it really was the only option for me.

When I went to join the military, I was turned away at the Military Entrance Processing Station the first time because I had lots of moles on my body (Dysplastic nevus syndrome). When the recruiter picked me up from my failed attempt, he told me something that would resonate with me for the rest of my life.

"You know you can get a waiver for your medical condition," he said.

"What's a waiver?" I asked.

A military medical waiver is a formal request to consider an applicant's suitability for service who, because of current or past medical conditions, does not meet medical standards. This would prove to be critically important to my military career and my entire life. When I earned my way into the enlisted commissioning program and applied for the special operations program, my vision wasn't good enough. I asked them if I could get a waiver, and they said, "Oh, yes, of course." I applied for the waiver and was accepted into the special operations pipeline.

Fast forward several more years, and I was in charge at the Deep Submergence Unit (DSU) in Coronado, California. I was trying to certify the new deep-submergence system, the Falcon pressurized rescue module. It was intended to replace the Mystic and the Avalon as the deep-submergence rescue and recovery asset for the US Navy. I learned that you could also get a "waiver" for things like pieces of equipment and testing, evaluation, and certification. This wound up being a crucial piece of information. When I was transferred to Special Operations Command in Tampa, Florida, I learned that I was now the Engineering program manager for a dry combat submersible. Part of my job was to develop waivers for the next dry combat submersible. The concept of waivers will become important later.

Being in the military is unlike a normal job in that the shared experience in traumatic situations sets us apart, along with our almost necessary dark sense of humor. Military guys are weird. For instance, we will pick on one another mercilessly, literally make fun of and put each other down, but we will fiercely and vigorously defend our buddy against any non-military person who crosses them.

When I was in Coronado, one of my old friends was Ed Winters, a two-star Admiral who was in command of Special Warfare Command when I was in charge at DSU as a Lieutenant Commander and Commander. Even though he was less than a mile away, I only knew him loosely, and that is to say that I knew him as the old guy who used to kayak and scuba dive by himself. We were friendly, but not close. When I transferred to Special Operations Command after my DSU tour, he was already stationed there. He and I then rekindled our friendship, becoming close enough to take weekly bike rides together every Wednesday.

He needed help moving out of base housing upon his retirement, and when he did, he asked all of his "friends" to come help him. I showed up, along with Admiral Bill McRaven and then-Lieutenant General Brad Heithold. Just imagine… Ed is a two-star Admiral, Bill is a four-star Admiral, and Brad is a three-star General. Together, there are nine stars and me moving Ed out of his house on MacDill Air Force Base. Let's just say that we did some drinking, and I did a lot of the moving. Hahaha.

After 27 years, 8 months, and 19 days of active-duty Naval service, I decided to end my service to the country. Leading up to this decision, I was struggling with my fourth bout of skin cancer and a seemingly ungrateful "Uncle Sam" who wanted me to move and become a geographical bachelor, leaving my family in Tampa while I went to do a tour in Washington, DC. I opted to stop working for my Uncle Sam.

Upon retirement from US Special Operations Command, I went through the standard identity crisis common to most military people. After 28 years of active-duty Navy service, you strongly identify with your rank; the rank is you. You are that person because that's all you've ever known. I had to do some deep (pun intended) soul-searching to figure out what my next intended job, position, or title would be, and how I would view myself. The one thing I missed most after retirement from the military was my "buddies," …that camaraderie and sharing of time.

When I was riding bikes with Ed every Wednesday morning, we would talk about the problems with the community. TBI and PTSD were rampant, and, at the time, we were losing 22 service members and veterans per day to suicide. I was already in school for my PhD and starting my research on TBI. He wanted me to help Admiral McRaven. I was asked to sit on a new initiative called the Preservation of the Force and Family (POTFF). Its goal was to help service members and their families. I gladly accepted, and it was a great honor to sit on that committee.

One of the problems that I found was that the people at POTFF were very much interested in "talking" to service members. Their main tenet at the time was talk therapy and psychology or psychiatry treatments. In my humble opinion, they did not understand military culture, and were unable to address service members' problems.

If they had taken the time to understand how people in the military think, they might have been able to come up with a better way to help them. Service members like to be part of the solution, not part of the problem. For example, imagine you told a tier-one operator that they were no longer part of the solution...You inform them that they are now part of the problem. But don't worry, you have a TBI, and we're going to take care of you. During my tenure on the POTFF, I saw too many service members diagnosed with a TBI who take their own lives. I went to Admiral McRaven, and I discussed my observation and opinion; and I will never forget the words he said to me: "Permission granted, Aquanaut... fix the problem."

One Friday, we were tracking an operator who was sent to San Antonio to be assessed for a TBI. The group got together and discussed his possible diagnosis. At the time, I assumed somebody was watching him, staying by his side in case he needed help. When you assume, you make an ass out of you and me, but still, I assumed. This man was diagnosed with a TBI and promptly went back to his government-furnished hotel room and shot himself. The Monday morning after we heard the news, we circled around and did a post-mortem discussion of the situation. When we looked at all the circumstances, I believed these smart people on the team knew, or should have known, that in our military culture, suicide would seem almost mandatory after a TBI diagnosis.

Warriors, operators, and doers never want to be part of the problem. We don't want to burden anybody. We don't want anybody wiping our behind or being upset because they now have to push us around in a wheelchair. There's also a very critical loss of residual self-image. We have a vision of us being young, invincible, and invisible. We all know this is not a healthy path to take, but nonetheless, it is a path we often take. We understand this, but we see it as necessary in order to be the do-gooders of the world. We envision ourselves as helpers or doers, people who like to get things done. To sideline any one of those people is tantamount to making them worthless or useless. You have to understand, when you diagnose somebody with that problem, unless you are there to help them, counsel them, hold them, and give them value pointed towards either a cure or a new normal, they are going to continue to perform this horrible, permanent solution to what may very well be a temporary problem.

That is, kind of, what got me started on my way to helping people with TBIs. My simple premise was that I wanted to start helping increase cerebral blood flow and support people with TBI using hyperbaric oxygen. As you can see from my personal account, it did not work fully. I was working on the flawed premise of doing one thing at a time.

It was time to go back to school and get my "learn on." By this point, I was emboldened to persevere in the face of any adversity because I was not a normal college student. I was a mid-40-year-old retired Naval officer, and many of the Professors were near my age. I still had this "waiver" mentality. When they told me I had to take the Graduate Record Exam (GRE), I said, "The GRE is a measure of your aptitude for completing graduate school; I can guarantee you with a hundred percent assurance that I can do that because I already have a master's degree in astronautical engineering." They insisted, and I said there has to be a waiver. I pushed back, and they let it go. They allowed me to enter a PhD program in biomedical engineering. When they asked me to take yet another statistics course, I pushed back, and I said my master's degree was in statistical orbital determination; I do not want to take that course... boom ...waiver.

Suffice it to say that the term "waiver" is and was etched into my memory as a good thing., Rules are rules ... but rules are made to be broken if you can break them the correct way. That laid the groundwork for all my research from then on.

I entered the world of fixing TBI with a single simplistic assumption: the system is broken and needs to be fixed. I learned the rules of the medical evaluation system and learned what was wrong with it, and then I decided that I was going to file for a waiver or find a way around it. Why? Because the current system isn't and wasn't working. The old club had millennia to figure out how to fix TBI. I was going to approach it differently.

That certainly started me on my way to try to figure out a new form of healing, but even I got pigeonholed into the "old way" of doing things. I was on the drug company model for testing and evaluating drug efficacy. The way that I was taught was a scientific process. Through the scientific process, you make steps such as observation and forming a null hypothesis, and then changing one variable at a time. That is to say, the way to discover what is happening, you may only have one intervention point at a time. That, I believe, is the fundamental flaw in current research methodology. Time for a waiver!

My life's journey, from a challenging childhood to a naval career and now academia, has been defined by resilience and a refusal to accept barriers. The waiver mentality, born from necessity, taught me to navigate rules creatively, whether in military service, personal relationships, or research. This mindset drives my mission to improve TBI treatment by challenging outdated systems to find solutions that honor the strength of those I serve.

CHAPTER THREE

Why is the healthcare system broken?

"All you need is a tincture of time."

BLUF – They literally told me those words. "All you need is a tincture of time." This chapter explores flaws in the pharmaceutical industry model as well as the double-edged sword of scientific testing... in short... why medicine is broken. It details some ways to fix it, but this is a bigger deal than Big Medicine will work on.

Somewhere between Aristotle, Galileo Galilei, and Sir Francis Bacon, we have lost our way in the observational method of science. We have developed and morphed our scientific method into a drug company model that is conspicuously devoid of any external thought of an overdetermined system. The human body is an overdetermined system, meaning that there are too many variables to control and not enough "knows" to solve the problem. We need to change the way we do science.

Medical doctors are often not scientists. They often use their white coats to inculcate fear. "Listen to me, or you could die." Much akin to "my best friend's sister's boyfriend's brother's girlfriend heard from a guy who knows a kid who's going with the girl who saw Ferris pass out at 31 Flavors last night." I believe they are not completely misinformed, but certainly they are myopic.

The researchers (who are scientists) who have realized this have been shamed and pushed aside, labeled conspiracy theorists or heretics. But the American public is sick of the white coat and the drug companies' death grip on our health! In this chapter, I will detail why we need a different way forward.

The pharmaceutical industry, often termed "Big Pharma," is a cornerstone of modern healthcare, developing drugs that address a wide range of medical conditions. However, its for-profit model, coupled with systemic flaws in the scientific process, raises profound ethical and practical concerns, fostering an over-reliance on medications in the United States and globally. I critically examined how the industry's structure, compounded by the limitations of scientific testing, undermines public health. The scientific method's reductionist approach, while rigorous, often fails to capture the complexity of human health.

The pharmaceutical industry's for-profit framework prioritizes financial returns over patient welfare, eroding trust in healthcare. Pharmaceutical companies focus on high-margin drugs for prevalent conditions, neglecting diseases with smaller market potential. "Evergreening" is a process wherein drug companies make minor drug modifications to extend patents. Evergreening delays affordable generic drugs. For instance, a 2020 JAMA analysis showed insulin prices in the U.S. increased by 200% from 2007 to 2018, despite no significant therapeutic advancements.[5]

---

[5] Anderson. (August 2024).

Here are just a few of the problems with Big Pharma:

- They continually mark up prices
- They pay for competitors to stay out of the market
- They spend billions of dollars on lobbying and marketing
- They have a monopoly on the market

Big Pharma shapes medical practice through funding and incentives. In 2020, Big Pharma paid physicians two billion dollars in gifts, consulting fees, and travel expenses.[6] It seems obvious that physicians receiving pharmaceutical payments would be more likely to prescribe brand-name drugs rather than generics, even when evidence supports equivalent efficacy. Why would physicians be allowed to receive these types of payments? Direct-to-consumer advertising, permitted only in the U.S. and New Zealand, drives demand for specific drugs, often bypassing clinical necessity, and marketing reinforces the general public's belief that they need to be on a pill. The commercials are often made sexy, fun, and appealing for most any drug.

The goal of research funding by for-profit companies is maximizing income to shareholders. Studies have found that companies may selectively fund trials on drugs that they consider to be superior to the competition.[7] Researchers paid by Big Pharma have at the very least an appearance of impropriety and a lack of objectivity. The "bias" that a researcher has should always be noted in their research. Researchers must report where their money comes from. In my opinion, when a drug company funds research for that drug company to profit

---

[6] Newham. (May 2024).

[7] Breault. (2020).

from… everyone in the room can see it is, at the very least, a perceived conflict of interest.

Publication bias undermines scientific integrity, with unfavorable trial results often withheld. In the research industry, we call this "cherry picking" your data. For example, a 2008 New England Journal of Medicine study on selective serotonin reuptake inhibitors (SSRIs) revealed that 94% of published trials reported positive results, while unpublished trials were more likely to show negative outcomes.[8] Further, to get pharmaceuticals through the FDA, drug companies must conduct testing, but those results are often sealed until it is time for a lawsuit. I believe we need more independent researchers focused on reporting the true data, not just information that supports a hypothesis.

Pharmaceutical companies exploit regulatory pathways like the FDA's Accelerated Approval. Many of the drugs approved in this manner lacked clinical benefit in follow-up studies. Notably, many antibiotics receive FDA clearance despite inappropriate manipulation of data analysis to enable a favored result. Furthermore, the "publish or perish" culture further incentivizes such practices. I have found myriad statistical errors in papers. It is important to check the bias of every single researcher and see where they get their money.

Medical insurance companies, operating as for-profit entities, prioritize financial outcomes over patient health. This is systemic and blatantly obvious to even the most casual of observers. Practitioners prescribe per their medical license and ability. Then a bean counter at the insurance office denies due to… whatever reason or issue they have with the provider or

[8] Fitzpatrick. (February 2010)

the service. According to recent research by the Kaiser Family Foundation, insurers of qualified health plans (QHPs) sold on HealthCare.gov denied 19% of in-network claims in 2024. The most common reasons cited by insurers in 2024 included "Other" [reason not listed] at 36%, followed by administrative reasons at 25%. Nine percent of denials were for lack of prior authorization or referral.[9] To me, these denials are tantamount to insurance companies practicing medicine without a license.

There is an insurance coverage pandemic. This profit-driven model leads to delays or denials of essential care, exacerbating health disparities. I know from my own personal experience with my father's condition that insured patients with chronic conditions face higher out-of-pocket costs. Unlike physicians, who are trained to prioritize patient welfare, insurance companies are corporations beholden to a board of directors. They may be interested in your "health" on a tertiary level, but with that priority conflict, they cannot be a healthcare company.

The scientific method is one of the most important discoveries of the last 400 years. The process we know today was first outlined by Francis Bacon as the inductive reasoning method. The scientific process involves core steps such as making an observation, asking a question based on that observation, conducting background research to understand what is already known, forming a testable hypothesis, designing and conducting an experiment to test the hypothesis, analyzing the data from the experiment, and finally, drawing a conclusion and communicating the results to others.

The scientific method underpins evidence-based medicine through structured clinical trials in four phases.

---

[9] Long. (March 2026).

Clinical Trial Phases

Phase	Description
Phase I	Assesses safety and dosage in small groups (20–100 participants)
Phase II	Evaluates efficacy and side effects in larger cohorts (100–300 participants)
Phase III	Confirms effectiveness via randomized controlled trials (RCTs) with thousands of participants
Phase IV	Monitors long-term effects post-market

The clinical trial process helps ensure drugs meet safety and efficacy standards through double-blind, placebo-controlled trials. However, its reductionist nature and commercial pressures reveal significant vulnerabilities. Case in point, there exists no double-blind randomized placebo-controlled trial that emphatically states that cigarettes cause cancer. ZERO… NOT ONE. That is because you cannot ethically administer such a controlled study. Does that mean cigarettes are good? Not in my opinion, but the fact is there are no studies which say they cause cancer. Further, the scientific method, while rigorous, is undermined by its implementation within a profit-driven system and its inherent limitations.

The scientific method isolates one variable at a time to ensure precision, but this approach often fails to capture the complexity of human health. Think of it this way: a tree requires a balanced combination of water, sunlight, and nutrients to thrive… too much of one element, like water, can kill it. If we were using the same scientific testing method that the pharmaceutical industry relies on, it would isolate each element without regard to the tree's complex needs or its environment. It would lead to absurd conclusions such as "water kills plants." As you can see, this method is profoundly flawed.

Similarly, clinical trials focus on single variables, neglecting other co-occurring conditions and genetic variability. The conventional, narrow approach to clinical trials, for the sake of simplicity, is a form of reductionism, producing results that are not generalizable to the broader population. Time and time again during COVID, we saw the most affected populations being the elderly, yet they were often excluded from trials, limiting the generalizability of the results. This approach overlooks the holistic needs of patients, leading to drugs that perform well in controlled settings but fail in real-world contexts. It may work for some people, but as we have seen over the last few thousand years, we are not winning the TBI pandemic! It is apparent that drugs are not the answer.

Drug development can cost billions of dollars and take 10–15 years.[10] These costs drive high drug prices, limiting access, with novel cancer therapies costing ridiculous amounts. Long timelines delay life-saving drugs, particularly for terminal conditions; regardless of the time it takes for the drugs to be produced or the cost, they should not be the permanent intervention. Ultimately, your body may need some drug to overcome a present issue or concern, but reliance upon drugs is not the preferred method of wellness today.

[10] Möhrle. (July 2024).

The focus on drug development marginalizes non-pharmacological interventions. There is no one paying a researcher to study gym attendance versus a pill as it relates to diabetes. This bias fosters medication dependency, sidelining preventive approaches. Often, these modifications and lifestyle changes are "thrown in" as a last resort, which leads to poor outcomes. Early non-pharmacological interventions should be considered, with a focus on lifestyle changes. Living better can make you better. No one needs a double-blind, randomized, placebo-controlled trial to tell me that eating well is good for me. I know intuitively that interventions should not be a last-ditch effort to get better; rather, they should be the way I live.

Physicians, constrained by time and industry influence, increasingly focus on conditions rather than patients. I believe these practitioners are victims of their own system. Time constraints and electronic health record demands reduce patient interaction, leading to a "checkbox" approach. I have had times where I needed to stop a physician who was halfway out the door to get them to answer my questions. I am sure many of you have seen or experienced something similar. Direct-to-consumer advertising exacerbates this, encouraging patients to seek drugs for specific diagnoses.

Daniel Kahneman is a psychologist best known for his work on the psychology of judgment and decision-making, as well as behavioral economics. In his book *Thinking, Fast and Slow*, for which he was awarded the 2002 Nobel Memorial Prize in Economic Sciences along with Vernon L. Smith, Kahneman outlines two systems humans use to make decisions. These are named system one and system two.

Decision Making Systems

Characteristic	System One	System Two
Speed	Fast-thinking system	Slower thinking system
Doubt and Certainty	Not prone to doubt; suppresses ambiguity; favors certainty	Capable of doubt, maintaining incompatible possibilities simultaneously
Function	Spontaneously constructs coherent stories	Reasoning

In this wonderful book, Kahneman uses what's called an "anchoring event" to illustrate how system one thinking works. He asks what year George Washington became president. The "anchoring event" that comes up is the Declaration of Independence and the ensuing war, which comes up in 1776. Most people estimate Washington became president around 1777 or sometime shortly after. System one estimates based on the anchoring event. But that is flawed thinking because Washington did not become president until 1789. System one does not allow for slower, more methodical reasoning.

System one thinking is the problem in TBI treatment. We know that everything the medical community has tried for the past several thousand years has had little to no impact on TBI. In system one thinking, there is no room for human nature or complexity; everyone must fit into the same cookie-cutter shape. This disregard for human complexity is one of the biggest problems with medicine right now! The medical community doesn't have a true cure for TBI; therefore, they tell us we only need a "tincture of time." I am not trying to beat up physicians. This is a difficult problem, but we can do something about it.

Think back a few pages to the phases of clinical trials and the number of participants in a study. Researchers are trying to achieve certain numbers so they can justify their "drug" or intervention as fitting a cookie-cutter size. Researchers are trying to look at a microcosm and apply it on a grand scale for everyone! Every person is different, and every person gets through a problem differently. There is a widespread misunderstanding of randomness, particularly when it comes to Healing TBI. There is no one-size-fits-all cure for anyone, and that is what makes it hard.

Let us do a case in point. You meet a PhD who is a professor. Your immediate assumption is that the person is very responsible. However, your practical experience tells you they left their shoes at your house and went home barefoot. The halo effect refers to the tendency to form many positive impressions about a person even though we know very little about that person. This is clearly system one knowledge. Again, we are just trying to fit people into cookie-cutter molds. With healing TBIs, the need for variation and individuality is the most important thing, so if you are struggling with your traumatic brain injury, perhaps it is because you have been placed in a cookie-cutter mold.

Humans are pattern seekers, and we should believe in a coherent world in which we can heal a TBI. Humans tend to try to make sense of chaos; the randomness of what works and what does not is difficult to understand, so we try to put things into little packages. Doctors appear to be too quick to perceive order, causality, and randomness. I opine it is their cognitive illusion. Fixing and helping is their job, their purpose, and the reason they went to medical school. The problem is that providers assume they know what caused someone's TBI, but how can we determine the true cause of TBI if providers are unable or unwilling to open the patient's head and take a look inside? We do not know causality for certain, and providers are speculating at best.

There is no admission of guilt for the failure of the medical community. No justice for those who have not been given hope. There has been no accountability for those in charge who smugly say there is no answer or you just need a tincture of time. No apology issued. This is all systemic hubris.

The medical community has betrayed our trust and taken away our hope. A "stain on the white coat" is becoming increasingly apparent. I believe doctors' egos get in their way. They are looking for evidence, as they should; however, the problem is they cloak themselves in the evidence., but the evidence is not their shield or their sword. Now, trust me when I tell you that I seek a healthy balance: I understand that a Google search, or even an AI meta search, is not equivalent to a medical degree, but that does not mean we should extinguish hope when evidence does not provide all of the answers .

Normal life should not be medicalized. TV and online ads market prescriptions for conditions like mild anxiety to our children. This mental health awareness movement is demonizing "pill shaming" and normalizing the use of medications. This is a propaganda plan with the express intent to leave the public reliant upon meds. "Do no harm" is the Hippocratic Oath, but doctors will offer "a tincture of time;" harm is being down by waiting. It is now common for TBI sufferers to be on some sort of medicine, but it is not healthy for the long-term. Short-term interventions are, in my opinion, possibly necessary depending on your situation, but the long-term solution for you to be on a pill seems like the exception rather than the rule. Further, direct-to-consumer (TV and radio) advertising undermines informed decision-making, as patients demand advertised drugs without understanding risks. Finally, the shift to condition-centered care reduces physicians' ability to understand patients' broader health context.

In science or research, we know that if we are doing things wrong, we are not getting the right result. If we remove all the other variables, what is left must be the truth. The truth is we have yet to find a cure for TBI, so at this point we have little left to do but to abandon the way that we have gone at it to start with a different premise and move forward from there.

To address these issues, the following reforms are proposed:

1. Promote non-pharmacological research. This should be the first point of intervention. Increase funding for lifestyle interventions.
2. Regulate industry practices with an independent organization responsible to the public. Enforce transparency in trial data and cap drug prices.
3. Enhance real-world evidence. Use real-world post-market data to make our trial results more applicable to everyday people.
4. Empower patients by expanding health literacy programs to counter direct-to-consumer advertising. We should not allow direct-to-consumer marketing for drugs, but we should interventions such as exercise and healthy living through marketing by public service announcements.

5. Reform regulatory frameworks and strengthen post-approval monitoring to ensure clinical benefit. For instance, go back and check efficacy, and if the drug or intervention fails in the full population, remove that drug from the shelf and ban it.
6. Reduce the research-to-practice gap by implementing strategies like:
   - Fostering collaborative research networks. Foster open-access platforms for sharing interim findings.
   - Streamline regulatory pathways. Expand adaptive trial designs to accelerate approvals without compromising safety.
   - Incentivize innovation adoption. Physicians are required to take continuing medical education credits regularly. If we fund those who adopt new research and implement it, we will create early adopters. Address the "not invented here" syndrome (the tendency to reject ideas or solutions from external sources) by funding incentives for cross-institutional collaboration.
7. Reform insurance models. Shift insurance incentives toward preventive care and patient outcomes.
8. Encourage holistic medicine. Increase training and time allocation for patient-centered care.
9. Promote wellness by offering lower healthcare costs for those who consistently take actions that benefit them from a health perspective.

The pharmaceutical industry's profit-driven model, coupled with the limitations of scientific testing, creates a flawed medical system. The scientific method's reductionist approach, likened to overwatering a tree, fails to capture the complexity of human health, while the maxim "science wins over bullshit, but what works ... works" underscores the value of practical outcomes. Researcher bias, driven by Big Pharma funding and the "publish or perish" culture, compounds issues like the 17-to-23-year research-to-practice gap. This gap in knowledge is unprecedented and getting bigger. As a society, we are more connected but less confident in the information we are provided with. We need a trusted platform from our government, responsible to the people. Finally, I believe for-profit insurance companies prioritize profit over health, exacerbating inequities. Supported by evidence from science, nature, and JAMA, this chapter calls for reforms to prioritize patient welfare, promote holistic care, and reduce delays in translating research to practice. Practical outcomes often outpace rigid scientific dogma, but I believe in the proverb, "science wins over bullshit, but what works ... works."

CHAPTER FOUR

Trying to heal – Creating a Multifaceted Approach as the Test Patient.

"When life gives you lemons ... learn to like lemons."

BLUF – This chapter chronicles my approach of blending personal experience with scientific rigor to offer a general guide for others navigating TBI recovery. These therapies could help and, most importantly,...will not hurt. This is a scientific approach to holistic ...not prescriptive... care, designed to get you off every drug, leading to a healthier life.

While I am not a medical doctor nor does this book provide medical advice, I maintain an educated opinion as I have contributed to medicine through my work and scientific research in the field of TBI. I also take my own healthcare seriously. This chapter specifically talks about treatments and protocols. It is important to work with myriad providers, as I did, and establish a treatment that could work for you. In my experience, I found that stacking different kinds of therapies offered the best results. Based upon the plant analogy and out of necessity to my previously discussed "timeline," I had to try everything and ultimately try it all at the same time.

After my accident, I found myself trapped in a mind that no longer functioned as it once did. The cognitive fog, emotional volatility, and physical pain were relentless reminders of the accident that had upended my life. As a biomedical engineer and clinical researcher, I refused to accept the conventional narrative that TBI recovery plateaus after a year. Instead, I embarked on a journey to explore off-label therapies, stacking them in a synergistic protocol to rebuild my brain and reclaim my life. In this chapter, I will explain my therapeutic journey and what worked for me.

Trauma-Focused Cognitive Behavioral Therapy

The first therapy I implemented was Trauma Recovery Intervention Protocol (TRIP). I was initially skeptical. I had always viewed therapy as an exploration of past relationships or social dynamics, but TRIP was different. TRIP is a neurological disconnect therapeutic intervention. This protocol was designed to allow my brain to be distracted while the amygdala allows the separation of the event and the emotions attached to the event, disconnecting without sharing the details of the traumatic event. Evidence has been collected from active-duty personnel, veterans, police officers, and firefighters to demonstrate the efficacy of the intervention and was compiled by an independent licensed clinical psychologist. Each 60 to 90-minute session felt like a mental workout, exhausting yet empowering. Over 5 weeks, I noticed a shift: my anxiety lessened, and my ability to focus improved. For me, it was a cornerstone of recovery, providing a psychological foundation for the physiological interventions that followed.

- **Implementation**: Engage with a TRIP therapist specializing in trauma for weekly 60 to 90-minute sessions over 5 to 12 weeks. Focus on exposure-based techniques and cognitive restructuring to address trauma-related symptoms.

Hyperbaric Oxygen Therapy

Hyperbaric oxygen therapy (HBOT) became a pivotal component of my recovery. I was inspired by decades in the field, as well as scientific information from my research for my book The Art and Science of Hyperbaric Medicine (2024). HBOT involves breathing pure oxygen in a pressurized chamber. This increases oxygen solubility in plasma, allowing it to reach brain regions with impaired circulation post-TBI.

I used HBOT twice daily for 60 minutes per session. HBOT enhances cerebral blood flow and reduces neuroinflammation. It's important to carefully monitor the process to avoid excessive vasoconstriction. The sessions were transformative; I felt clearer and alert, and less fatigued. Over 40 sessions, I noticed improvements in memory and processing speed, as if my brain was slowly rewiring itself.

- **Implementation**: Use this treatment only under medical supervision. Administer HBOT at 1.5–2.0 ATA for 60 minutes, twice daily, for 20 to 40 sessions.

How and Why HBOT Works for TBI

The science behind HBOT is compelling, and I have gone to great lengths to study its effects on the human body (see my book: The Art and Science of Hyperbaric Medicine). By dissolving oxygen in plasma, HBOT bypasses hemoglobin-dependent transport, delivering oxygen to poorly perfused tissues. This was particularly critical for my brain, where microcirculatory damage from the injury had created pockets of hypoxia. Comprehending the mechanisms of action of HBOT is essential for practitioners, as it empowers them to apply the known Mechanisms of Action (MOAs) of approved indications across a broad spectrum of health concerns and goals. Although some indications may not be clinically proven through double-blind, placebo-controlled studies, practitioners can still make reasonable assumptions about the treatment's efficacy and conduct trials to observe its effects. The following is a list of MOAs to help in your understanding of how and why this treatment works as effectively as it does.

1. **Decreased Bubble Size (Boyle's Law):** Hyperbaric oxygen therapy reduces the volume of intravascular and tissue gas bubbles according to Boyle's Law, whereby increasing ambient pressure decreases bubble size. In the context of blast-induced traumatic brain injury, the rapid pressure wave from an explosion can generate micro-bubbles or gas emboli within the cerebral vasculature. These bubbles contribute to mechanical obstruction, endothelial damage, and secondary neuroinflammation. By reducing bubble volume, HBOT may decrease vascular obstruction, limit ischemic injury, and reduce the inflammatory cascade triggered by bubble-induced endothelial activation and leukocyte recruitment in neural tissue.
2. **Hyperoxygenation:** Hyperbaric oxygen significantly increases the partial pressure of oxygen dissolved in plasma, allowing oxygen to reach hypoxic tissues that

are poorly perfused due to edema, microcirculatory disruption, or vascular injury. In traumatic brain injury and spaceflight-associated physiological stress, this enhanced oxygen delivery can restore aerobic metabolism in marginally perfused brain regions, reduce anaerobic glycolysis, and support cellular energy production without relying solely on hemoglobin-bound oxygen.

3. **Reduced Lipid Peroxidation:** Hyperbaric oxygen therapy decreases lipid peroxidation of cell membranes by modulating reactive oxygen species and upregulating antioxidant defenses. In blast and impact traumatic brain injury, lipid peroxidation contributes to membrane damage, axonal injury, and propagation of neuroinflammation. By limiting oxidative damage to neuronal and glial membranes, HBOT may help preserve cellular integrity and reduce secondary injury cascades in the brain.
4. **Vasoconstriction with Improved Oxygenation:** Hyperbaric oxygen induces vasoconstriction while simultaneously increasing oxygen content in the blood. This combination reduces cerebral edema and intracranial pressure without compromising oxygen delivery to brain tissue. In neurotrauma and conditions involving cerebral swelling, this mechanism can help control vasogenic edema while maintaining adequate oxygenation, potentially mitigating secondary brain injury.
5. **Reduced Intravascular Leukocyte Adherence:** Hyperbaric oxygen reduces the adherence of leukocytes to the endothelium, thereby decreasing the release of proinflammatory mediators and reactive oxygen species

at sites of injury. In traumatic brain injury, excessive leukocyte activation contributes to blood-brain barrier disruption and neuroinflammation. By attenuating this response, HBOT may limit secondary inflammatory damage to neural tissue.

6. **Toxin Inhibition:** Hyperbaric oxygen inhibits the function of certain bacterial toxins and reduces the toxicity of carbon monoxide by accelerating its dissociation from hemoglobin and cytochrome oxidase. While primarily established in infectious and toxicological conditions, this mechanism may have relevance in polytrauma scenarios where bacterial contamination or systemic toxin release occurs alongside blast or impact injury.
7. **Enhanced Leukocyte Oxidative Killing:** Hyperbaric oxygen improves the oxidative killing capacity of leukocytes by increasing the availability of oxygen required for the respiratory burst. This mechanism enhances the immune system's ability to combat infection, which is particularly relevant in trauma patients who are at elevated risk of wound and systemic infections due to tissue damage and immune dysregulation.
8. **Antibiotic Synergy:** Hyperbaric oxygen acts synergistically with certain antibiotics, improving their efficacy against anaerobic and facultative organisms. In complex trauma involving contaminated wounds or osteomyelitis, this synergy can enhance infection control and support tissue recovery when used as an adjunct to standard antimicrobial therapy.

9. **Growth Factor Release** (Angiogenesis, Neurogenesis, and Mitogenesis): Hyperbaric oxygen stimulates the release of growth factors such as vascular endothelial growth factor (VEGF), platelet-derived growth factor, and others that promote angiogenesis, neurogenesis, and cellular proliferation. In traumatic brain injury, these effects may support neovascularization, neural repair, and functional recovery in damaged brain regions.
10. **Fibroblast Proliferation and Collagen Synthesis:** Hyperbaric oxygen enhances fibroblast proliferation and collagen deposition, which are essential for wound healing and tissue remodeling. In the context of trauma and surgical recovery, this mechanism supports the structural repair of damaged tissues and may aid in the resolution of chronic or non-healing wounds.
11. **Stem Cell Proliferation and Mobilization:** Hyperbaric oxygen promotes the proliferation and mobilization of stem cells, including hematopoietic and mesenchymal stem cells, from bone marrow into circulation. These cells can migrate to sites of injury and contribute to tissue repair, angiogenesis, and modulation of inflammation, offering a regenerative component to recovery from traumatic brain injury.
12. **Increased Reverse Transcriptase Activity:** Hyperbaric oxygen has been shown to increase reverse transcriptase activity, which may support DNA repair processes and cellular regeneration. This mechanism is thought to contribute to genomic stability and recovery from oxidative and radiation-induced DNA damage.

13. **Reduction of Cytokine Activity and Neuroinflammation:** Hyperbaric oxygen downregulates pro-inflammatory cytokines, including interleukin-6 (IL-6) and tumor necrosis factor-alpha, while modulating the overall inflammatory response. In traumatic brain injury and blast-related neurotrauma, excessive cytokine activity drives neuroinflammation, blood-brain barrier dysfunction, and secondary neuronal injury. By attenuating this inflammatory cascade, HBOT may reduce neuroinflammation and help preserve neurological function.[11]

Now that you know more about HBOT, we can move on to the other therapies that I tried during my recovery from TBI.

Structural Energetic Therapy (SET)

Structural Energetic Therapy (SET) helps to realign the body and the brain. Pain from normal military life exacerbated by a shoulder injury sustained during my accident was a constant reminder of my trauma, keeping my brain locked in a state of distress. The vagus nerve is a key regulator of the parasympathetic nervous system. Its job is to reinforce this feedback loop, signaling to my brain that I was still "injured" through the fact that the shoulder was still injured. It was a reminder of sorts. To address this, I turned to SET, a targeted massage technique that identifies musculoskeletal imbalances and tension "hotspots."

My SET sessions were revelatory. The therapist observed my posture and gait, pinpointing areas of tension in my neck and lower back. Breathwork sessions that emphasized

[11] Dituri. (2024).

diaphragmatic breathing produced an almost euphoric sense of release, akin to an out-of-body experience. Even with my 25 years of martial arts training and a third-degree black belt, I had never encountered anything so profound. The sacral-cranial component, involving gentle manipulation of the occipital lobe, was equally impactful. By slightly shifting the skull, the therapist enhanced CSF flow, thereby reducing circulation time and helping the brain repair itself. Each session left me deeply relaxed, with a newfound sense of physical and mental harmony.

- **Implementation**: Schedule weekly 60-minute SET sessions with a certified practitioner, focusing on breathwork and sacral-cranial massage. Practice daily diaphragmatic breathing to sustain benefits.

Neurofeedback Therapy

Neurofeedback Therapy is a way of training the brain to heal itself. Neurofeedback became a game-changer in my recovery. This therapy measures brainwave activity and provides real-time audio-visual feedback to train the brain toward optimal patterns. For TBI patients, neurofeedback targets dysregulated alpha and theta waves, improving attention, emotional regulation, and cognitive clarity.[12] My sessions, costing $6,000 out of pocket, were a significant investment, but the results were undeniable. After my accident, I struggled with certain deficits that made it difficult to focus, manage stress, and process complex research papers. After 20 sessions, I could process complex research papers again, a task that had been maddening post-TBI.

[12] Gray. (August 2017).

The system I used leveraged Pavlovian conditioning, rewarding my brain for producing desired wave patterns. Each 90-minute session felt like a mental recalibration, gradually restoring my ability to focus and manage stress. Inspired by the results, I invested $40,000 in a neurofeedback machine for my research clinic, ensuring access for others, particularly service members who couldn't afford such care. This therapy underscored the power of self-regulation, empowering me to take control of my brain's recovery.

- **Implementation**: Work with a trained clinician when attempting this treatment. Complete 20 to 40 neurofeedback sessions, with each session 60 to 90 minutes in length; I suggest using a QEEG-guided protocol tailored to individual brainwave deficits.

Brain Tap

Brain Tap is an over-the-counter meditation aid tool that wound up being my gateway to mindfulness. Meditation was challenging for me, a Type A personality accustomed to constant action. Brain Tap, a device that combines binaural beats, light therapy, and guided visualization, made meditation both accessible and transformative. By delivering dual auditory inputs (one to each ear) and emitting light patterns even with eyes closed, Brain Tap trains brainwaves to promote relaxation and focus.[13] The subliminal effect of processing two auditory streams simultaneously anchored me in the present, quieting my racing mind.

[13] Tang. (March 2015).

I used Brain Tap daily, selecting from 50 to 60 pre-programmed sessions targeting stress relief, cognitive enhancement, or sleep. Each 20-minute session felt like a mental reset, reducing cortisol and fostering neuroplasticity. For TBI patients, this tool is invaluable, particularly for those who find traditional meditation daunting. Brain Tap became a cornerstone of my routine, complementing the physiological benefits of other therapies. I termed it "meditation for people who don't like meditation."

- **Implementation**: Use Brain Tap for 20 to 30 minutes daily in a quiet, dimly lit space. Choose sessions aligned with specific goals, such as relaxation or cognitive focus.

Ice Bath Therapy

Ice Bath Therapy was one of the most unexpected yet transformative tools in my recovery. The idea struck me while driving past a sign advertising "ICE $5."

Taking an ice bath (in water between 32 and 50°F) can have two main effects:

- It may force or redirect blood to your brain, which increases the delivery of blood and oxygen (cerebral perfusion) to the brain tissue.
- It triggers the release of special healing proteins called cold shock proteins, which speed up your body's recovery process (Lieberman et al., 2019).

My first 5-minute session in 32°F water was grueling, but by focusing on controlled breathing, I pushed through the discomfort. The mental clarity and physical invigoration that followed were profound. It shocked me to learn this was a trend among biohackers and a lifestyle for many. Over time, I grew to love the process, incorporating 5 to 10-minute sessions 3 to 5 times weekly. The mental discipline required to endure the cold translated into greater emotional control, a critical asset for TBI recovery. There are many more benefits to ice bath therapy.[14]

Research shows that ice baths not only center your mind and steel your resolve, but they also boast a 13% increase in brown adipose tissue.[15] This is important because brown adipose tissue is the mitochondrial-dense fat, which is the "good fat." Further, the endorphin release is off the charts. It boasts somewhere between 200 to 250 times the endorphins normally released by pleasurable activities. Also, cold forces vasoconstriction and vasodilation. This means there is both an increase and decrease in blood flow, which increases nitric oxide synthase (NOS). NOS is a smooth muscle mediator which helps you open and close blood vessels, increasing or restricting blood flow. I have noticed profound reductions in my pain level. Ice baths purport to help with Alzheimer's disease as well, showing promise in diabetes.[16] This is clearly preliminary and small trials, but nonetheless compelling. RBM3 is also increased. RBM3 is a cold-induced RNA-binding protein and is involved in mRNA biogenesis and exerts anti-apoptotic effects; this means it preserves the cell. Brain-derived neurotrophic factor (BDNF), the lawn seed for the brain, is upregulated. Ice baths can also stimulate hormesis and enlarge the anterior

[14] See Appendix A

[15] Nedergaard. (August 2007).

[16] Tournissac. (April 2019).

mid-cingulate cortex, a brain region critical for attention, decision-making, and error detection.

- **Implementation**: Perform 3 to 10-minute ice baths at 32 to 50°F, 3 to 5 times weekly, focusing on diaphragmatic breathing. Gradually increase duration as tolerance improves from 3 to 10 minutes.

Brain Games

Brain games stimulate neuroplasticity. They can be computer-generated or paper-based. I chose brain games designed to challenge cognitive function. Platforms like Lumosity and CogniFit offered exercises targeting memory, attention, and problem-solving, stimulating neural adaptation.[17] Unlike mindless phone games, these tools felt productive, engaging my brain in ways that felt like physical exercise. Daily 15 to 30-minute sessions helped restore my ability to process complex information, a skill that had been severely impaired post-TBI.

I also started working more on mathematical games such as Sudoku and on complex mathematical challenges (i.e. starting at 0, adding 8, then subtracting 6, then adding 1, counting continually, and ending at 56.) This type of processing helped me maintain order in my brain. Another "fun" math game was to take a four-digit number and, in one-second intervals, add one to each of the digits, with this exercise continuing multiple times through a series of flashcards. When you do this, your pupils will dilate.

Something noteworthy is that if you multitask with these brain games, your gains are greater. That means if you both go

[17] Hardy. (September 2015).

for a brisk walk and have your friend quiz you on numbers, you are better off than just doing the numbers. Alternatively, if you are listening to an audiobook while working out and, every few minutes, you pause the book and make a conscious effort to recall the main points, you are helping your brain. Strive to multitask!

You can also try games like Sudoku, Chess, and crossword puzzles. For me, brain games were more than a cognitive workout; they were a reminder that my brain could adapt and grow, even after significant injury. This aligned with my emphasis on leveraging neuroplasticity to overcome TBI deficits. If you don't use it … you lose it.

- **Implementation**: Engage in daily 15 to 30-minute sessions using evidence-based brain training apps or some sort of thinking and processing systems that can be checked and measured, and which focus on memory and executive function tasks.

Life Coaching

Life Coaching helped me to navigate to a new normal. My life coach helped me navigate the cognitive and emotional challenges of TBI. He was like an emergency physician for the soul, guiding me to develop compensatory strategies for my visuospatial deficits. Post-TBI, my eyes were misaligned, reminiscent of childhood strabismus, making reading a nightmare. My coach taught me to prioritize tasks, manage my schedule, and address frustrations with practical solutions. His approach echoed the compensatory behaviors I had developed as a child, adapting to new challenges with resilience.[18]

[18] Seligman. (2005).

Weekly sessions transformed my outlook, helping me find balance and purpose. For TBI patients, such coaching is invaluable, bridging the gap between physical recovery and emotional well-being.

- **Implementation**: Schedule biweekly 60-minute sessions with a life coach trained in TBI recovery, focusing on goal-setting, stress management, and compensatory strategies.

Physical Therapy

Physical therapy was one of the most important therapies I tried. When I was in my car accident, not only did my head strike the window, but the impact of the crumpled door hurt my left shoulder. Physical therapy was critically important to my recovery. If you haven't read the book *The Body Keeps the Score*, by Bessel van der Kolk, you should. It explains how the trauma of physical actions reminds a person of their psychological and physiological failures. A person must heal their physical, physiological, and psychological viewpoints simultaneously; otherwise, they will remain in that reminder cycle.

- **Implementation**: Schedule a session weekly for approximately a month to eliminate, or at least reduce, certain physical. Make sure your physical fitness regimen includes physical therapy assignments as dictated by your provider.

Chiropractic Care

Chiropractic care may aid in healing TBI. There is some research showing that the adjustment of misaligned vertebrae (a condition known as subluxation) ensures optimal nerve communication. For TBI patients, this can reduce the strain on the brain's ability to coordinate bodily functions, leading to improvements in mobility and cognitive clarity.[19] By correcting subluxations, chiropractic care may improve cerebrospinal fluid flow and reduce neuroinflammation, indirectly supporting brain healing.[20] It also complements breathing techniques by reducing physical stress that hinders diaphragmatic breathing.

- **Implementation**: Seek a licensed chiropractor experienced in neurological conditions, scheduling 1 to 2 sessions weekly for adjustments targeting the cervical and thoracic spine. Combine with breathing exercises to maximize relaxation and recovery.

Nature Exposure and Grounding

Several studies have shown that exposure to nature enhances both psychological and physiological well-being.[21] Immersion in nature, particularly listening to birdsong, reduces stress and helps with neural regulation. Studies show forest soundscapes improve mood and cognitive function.[22] So, get off your phone and get outside.

- **Implementation**: Spend 30 to 60 minutes daily in green spaces (parks, forests), focusing on natural sounds like birdsong. Use noise-canceling headphones with recorded birdsong if outdoor access is limited, ideally in the morning to align with circadian rhythms (I prefer nature).

[19] Chun-Pu. (May 2022)..
[20] Amjad. (December 2025).
[21] Baquedano. (April 2026).
[22] Longman. (September 2025).

Grounding, or earthing, involves direct contact with the Earth (e.g., walking barefoot on grass) to absorb electrons, potentially reducing inflammation and improving healing.[23] Facing east to catch sunrise exposes you to natural light, regulating circadian rhythms, boosting serotonin, and improving sleep quality, critical for TBI recovery. These practices enhance mood and energy, supporting mental resilience.

- **Implementation**: Spend 20 to 30 minutes daily barefoot on natural surfaces (like grass or sand) and 10 to 15 minutes at sunrise facing east, ideally in a quiet outdoor setting. Combine with deep breathing to amplify benefits.

My therapeutic journey also included using a Bemer™ Mat, Hormone Modulation Therapy, Peptides, KAATSU Band Therapy, and Red-Light Therapy.

Pulsed Electromagnetic Field Therapy (PEMF)

Pulsed Electromagnetic Field Therapy (PEMF), such as that delivered by a Bemer™ brand mat delivers pulsed electromagnetic fields to stimulate cellular repair, reduce inflammation, and enhance blood flow. PEMF may support TBI recovery by improving mitochondrial function, reducing oxidative stress, and promoting neurogenesis, with studies suggesting benefits for neurological conditions like depression and chronic pain. It's non-invasive and can complement other therapies by optimizing cellular energy.

[23] Oschman. (March 2015)..

- **Implementation:** Consult a practitioner before use. Use a PEMF device like the Bemer™ mat for 15 to 30 minutes daily, selecting low-frequency settings (5 to 15 Hz). Place the mat under your head or body during sessions.

Red Light Therapy (RLT)

While evidence related to treatment of TBI is still developing, Red Light Therapy (RLT) enhances mitochondrial function, increases ATP production (adenosine triphosphate), and promotes cerebral blood flow, potentially aiding neuronal repair.[24] I used an RLT mat combined with a grounding mat, lying on them for 20 minutes daily. This warm and gentle stimulation was deeply relaxing, and I believe it contributed to reduced inflammation and improved mood. The grounding mat, by reducing systemic inflammation, may have amplified these benefits. For TBI patients, the low-risk, high-reward nature of RLT makes it an appealing complement to other therapies.

- **Implementation:** Perform daily 20-minute RLT sessions using a 660–850 nm mat, paired with a grounding mat. Ensure consistent exposure for cumulative benefits.

Shake Plate / Whole-Body Vibration (WBV) Therapy

Shake plate therapy, also called whole-body vibration (WBV) therapy, is delivered via a "shake plate" or vibrating platform and involves standing or performing exercises on a device that transmits mechanical vibrations (20–50 Hz) to stimulate muscles, bones, and neural pathways without high-impact stress. For TBI survivors, WBV can attenuate brain damage by reducing neuroinflammation, improving motor performance, and

[24] Hamblin. (November 2017).

enhancing coordination and behavioral control. There are preclinical models where vibrations promoted neuronal activity and reduced arousal-induced hyperactivity. It also boosts blood flow and Vascular Endothelial Growth Factor (VEGF), supporting angiogenesis and tissue repair, similar to exercise but with less physical strain, making it accessible for those with mobility limitations.

- **Implementation:** Perform daily for 10 minutes per day. Advanced techniques can include combining subtle bending and dips to include balancing exercises during the period. Ultimately two 10-minute periods seemed helpful for me.

Hormone Modulation Therapy and Peptides:
While drugs were not a center or core of my program, some pharmaceutical interventions for short periods of time may be necessary. For instance, I needed something to help me sleep, which allowed me to catch up on sleep and start the healing process. There should be an intention with ANY program to get off the pharmaceuticals as quickly as possible.

Hormone modulation, including peptide therapies like BPC-157 or Cerebrolysin, aims to restore hormonal balance and promote neuroprotection (see the drugs chapter for detailed discussion). TBI often disrupts the hypothalamic-pituitary axis, leading to deficiencies in growth hormone, testosterone, or other hormones critical for brain repair and mood regulation. Peptides like BPC-157 may enhance angiogenesis, reduce inflammation, and accelerate tissue healing, with animal studies showing improved recovery from brain trauma. Cerebrolysin, a neuropeptide preparation, has shown potential in improving cognitive outcomes post-TBI by supporting neuroplasticity and reducing oxidative stress.

- **Implementation:** Work with an endocrinologist or specialist experienced in peptide therapy and hormone therapy to assess hormone levels and administer off-label treatments. Dosing varies, and protocols must be individualized, with regular monitoring for side effects like hormonal imbalances.

KAATSU Band Therapy

KAATSU, or blood flow restriction (BFR) therapy, uses specialized cuffs to partially restrict blood flow during low-intensity exercise, mimicking the benefits of high-intensity training. This promotes muscle growth, strength, and growth hormone release, which can support TBI recovery by enhancing physical resilience and neuroprotection. BFR also increases VEGF and Nitric Oxide Synthase (NOS), improving cerebral blood flow and potentially aiding brain repair. For TBI survivors, KAATSU's low-impact nature is ideal for those with limited mobility.

- **Implementation:** Use FDA-approved KAATSU bands under professional guidance, applying them to arms or legs during light resistance exercises (e.g., 20–30% of max effort) for 15 to 20 minutes, 2 to 3 times weekly. Start with low pressure (100–150 mmHg) and adjust based on comfort and professional advice.

Lifestyle Changes

As a commitment to the healing process, I eliminated alcohol and tobacco use for the length of my recovery. I further limited caffeine intake to no more than two cups of coffee daily (both before noon) to help with sleep. I made sure all caffeine intake stopped by noon each day for the same reason. In the interest of adequate hydration, I consumed a minimum of one gallon of water each day before 6 pm. I made an agreement with myself to adhere to a sleep schedule of 8 hours each night. That meant that, short of necessity or emergency, I would not get out of bed during my designated sleep window, even if I was not asleep.

At first, I focused on simple movement, and later added the gym; at a minimum, I would walk three miles (6500 steps) twice a week. Most importantly, when you go to the gym, you need to vary your routine. Variety is your spice of life to increase cerebral blood flow and restore synaptic pathways. Not just weights or just cardio, but an ever-changing lineup of gym workouts that will force you to think and build new bridges. If your workouts are too easy, you may be getting too comfortable in whatever you're doing. You need to continually challenge yourself to grow. Critical to this process was an accountability buddy. I found that having someone at the gym or walking with me made excuses less frequent, and a routine easier to maintain.

As with many things in this book, I have discovered that the whole is greater than the sum of its parts. Stacking all these therapies: TF-CBT, HBOT, SET, neurofeedback, Physical therapy, chiropractic therapy, Brain Tap, RLT, ice baths, brain games, and life coaching helped me create a synergistic protocol that addressed the physical, psychological, and physiological dimensions of TBI. My journey taught me that recovery is multifaceted, requiring persistence and creativity. Don't give up. Keep doing something. Does some of this seem "woo woo?" Yes, it does. Will the "woo woo" hurt you? No, it will not. While some therapies lack large-scale randomized trials, their mechanistic plausibility and clinical efficacy make them powerful tools for TBI patients. By combining these interventions, I not only healed my brain but discovered a resilience I never knew I possessed. I encourage others to explore these options under the appropriate medical supervision, tailoring the protocol to their unique needs. Remember to seek low-cost options that have an impact.

CHAPTER FIVE

D.E.S.S.E.R.T.S.
(The Gut-Brain Axis in Traumatic Brain Injury)

"Why, sometimes I've believed as many as six impossible things before breakfast."

-Lewis Carroll, Alice's Adventures in Wonderland

BLUF – Diet, Exercise, Stress, Sleep, Repetitive Exposure to Toxins, and Sunlight exposure are so closely related that I cannot in good conscience write a chapter on one without speaking about the impact from all of them simultaneously on the human body. Simply put, a change in any one of these causes a corresponding change in the other.

The goal of this chapter is to work towards getting people off drugs for their TBI. I also want to educate the reader on what is going on inside the gut and the body as well as point out what we can do to fix it. Ultimately, we aim for people to obtain all their nutrition naturally from the food they eat.

I opine that the real weapons of mass destruction in the diet of Americans are: highly or ultra-processed foods; pesticide-sprayed produce; high fructose corn syrup; over-sugared, low-fiber, food-like substances with "natural flavors;" and hot food stored in plastic containers. I do not consider those real food, so I call them "foods." These types of "foods" provide little to no nutrition. I have learned that what we eat, when we eat, and how much and what we drink, are key contributors to healing. This ever-changing lineup of diet, breathing techniques, and fluid intake affects the hypothalamic-pituitary-adrenal (HPA) axis, a communication system between the brain, the pituitary gland, and the adrenal glands. You will see how the HPA is crucial for your body's stress management.

It is likely time to overhaul your diet, whether you have had a TBI or not. The typical American diet is horrifying and horrible for us. I have struggled with gut issues for a while. From my time in the military, I got to eat new and "interesting" foods in foreign lands, which did not help my problems. In my research, I have learned a lot, including that your gut starts at your mouth and ends at your anus. All the parts in between are integral and should be taken care of, including brushing your teeth. There is so much to get into with respect to the gut and related issues; I am truly barely scratching the surface when it comes to gut health. The methods herein may be somewhat difficult to implement, but they are better than the pain in the ass (literally) of dealing with stomach and wellness issues.

This chapter explores the gut-brain axis as it relates to TBI, focusing on gastrointestinal dysfunction. I have found dietary, lifestyle, and integrative interventions to optimize TBI recovery. By prioritizing gut health, individuals can reduce inflammation, stabilize mood, and enhance cognitive restoration, allowing for a holistic approach to TBI management.

What is Happening in the Gut (The Science of the Gut and TBI): The gut, often called the "second brain" for its extensive neural network and production of neurotransmitters such as serotonin, is critical for modulating neuroinflammation and supporting recovery after TBI. The gut-brain axis is a dynamic communication network linking the gastrointestinal (GI) tract and the central nervous system, integrating neural, hormonal, and immunological signals to regulate digestion, mood, and cognition. We know that TBI disrupts this axis, triggering systemic inflammation and complicating recovery. Chronic inflammation impairs neurotransmitter signaling, contributing to mood disorders, cognitive deficits, and behavioral changes.

TBI compromises the intestinal lining, necessitating repair to reduce neuroinflammation. In my experience, gut healing typically takes 2 to 6 months: mild cases resolve in 2 to 3 months, while severe cases require 4 to 6 months or more. (See Appendix A for more information on the science of the gut and TBI).

Diet, Sleep, Stress, and Exercise

Sleep is one of the most fundamental needs in the human body. TBI sufferers have some of the greatest problems with sleep, whether they are derived from physical discomfort, physiological changes, or psychological issues. This book is not an all-encompassing treatise on sleep, but it is advisable to heed the advice herein to ameliorate sleep issues so you can heal. Seek some real sleep guidance from a professional if you still cannot sleep.

Diets and gym memberships seldom work alone, but everyone tries them. Every other day, the FDA or physicians change the "what is bad for me" food, and we never know the truth about good or bad foods. As we age, muscle loss increases; everyone tends to lose muscle mass as they age. Building muscle is one of the best things you can do to positively impact your nervous system. While I cannot teach you about all the dietary changes and exercises that can help reduce muscle loss as you grow older, I hope this motivates you to dive deeper into an exercise routine. Ultimately, fat acts like an endocrine organ and secretes hormones which can promote clot formation. Your excess weight will contribute acutely to your pain and increase the healing time for your brain.

Stress is the physical and emotional reaction we experience from challenges in life. Stress causes a great deal of the stomach issues TBI sufferers experience. But stress and worry are for nothing because we cannot control most of the things we worry about. Below are several stress management techniques that I have found helpful on my road to recovery. Common negative effects of stress include mental health issues like anxiety and sleep problems.

Science Blah Blah Blah…What Can We Do About It?

- Eat fiber and an anti-inflammatory diet to reduce inflammation and help with recovery.[25]
- Because HBOT reduces systemic inflammation, its use may enhance these mechanisms.
- Hydration supports gut health, microbial balance, and toxin clearance and is absolutely crucial for TBI recovery.[26] Hydration maintains the gut microbiota.[27] Gut massage can restore motility and microbial balance.[28]
- Diet profoundly influences the gut-brain axis, shaping microbial composition, inflammation, and neurological outcomes. Processed foods, high in sugars and trans fats,

[25] Yu. (January 2019)

[26] Detailed guidance regarding the intersection of proper hydration and traumatic brain injuries is located within Appendix A..

[27] Sato. (May 2024).

[28] Liu. (December 2025).

promote dysbiosis and inflammation, worsening TBI outcomes.[29]

- Whole foods, rich in fiber, polyphenols, and fermented products, support microbial diversity and anti-inflammatory pathways.
- Eat fermented foods, like sauerkraut, kimchi, and yogurt. These foods introduce probiotics and prebiotics, which help to restore microbial balance post-TBI.[30] The science behind fermented foods is fascinating.[31]
- Avoid microplastics found in plastic food packaging.
- Practice mindfulness in your everyday life. Meditation, a cornerstone of mindfulness, is a scientifically supported method for reducing stress and fostering resilience by influencing these neural networks.
- More guidance about diet, hydration, and mindfulness is in Appendix A

Below, we detail dietary strategies, emphasizing hydration, fermented foods, intestinal repair, and strategic shopping: An anti-inflammatory diet, featuring fruits, vegetables, nuts, seeds, and omega-3 fatty acids like salmon, reduces neuroinflammation and supports brain repair. The Mediterranean diet, as practiced by Sardinian centenarians, features olive oil, fish, whole grains, and vegetables, enhancing microbial diversity and SCFA production. These diets stabilize the gut-brain axis and can aid TBI recovery.[32]

[29] Shaito. (June 2020).
[30] Berding. (March 2021).
[31] See fermented foods section in Appendix A.
[32] Krakovski. (September 2022).

Some research supports the ketogenic diet to help stimulate your brain in recovery. This diet is high in fats and low in carbohydrates, inducing ketosis and altering microbial composition. Ketosis is a form of hormesis. This is not just a diet but a means to increase your metabolic flexibility.[33] It is meant to stimulate your brain and not meant to be a forever diet, but the brain's preferred source of fuel is ketones over glucose or sugar.

Dietary needs vary by metabolism, genetics, and culture. The key is prioritizing whole, unprocessed foods tailored to individual needs. TBI patients should shop the grocery store's perimeter, where fresh produce, lean proteins, and minimally processed dairy are found, avoiding central aisles' ultra-processed foods (e.g., chips, sodas, packaged snacks). Processed foods contain additives, like emulsifiers, that disrupt gut barriers, leading to inflammation and disease.[34] It may help to eliminate gluten, certain kinds of dairy products, processed foods, and additives.

Strategic Shopping Guidance:

- Fresh Produce: Chóose organic leafy greens, berries, and avocados to minimize pesticide exposure. Organic options reduce chemical residues that worsen TBI-related inflammation. Be sure to wash fruit prior to refrigerating to remove dirt, wax, or any other crud they put on fruit prior to shipping.
- Proteins: Foods like fresh wild-caught salmon are rich in omega-3s. Poultry or lentils are great sources as well. Avoid processed meats like sausages or anything that

[33] Erdman. (2011).

[34] Hogenboom. (February 2026).

contains preservatives, which can impair gut function. Omega-3s and polyphenols strengthen gut barriers.[35]

- Minimally Processed Dairy: Select the unsweetened yogurt or kefir with live cultures, avoiding sugary or flavored yogurts that feed pathogens.
- Whole Grains and Nuts: If you choose to eat grains, look for quinoa, brown rice, or raw nuts, avoiding prepackaged snacks with artificial flavors.

Reading labels is the next great thing in your life. Simply put, avoid things you don't understand, as well as natural flavors, artificial sweeteners, and hydrogenated oils. This approach minimizes dietary toxins, supports microbial balance, and enhances nutrient absorption, all critical for the TBI patient's sensitive gut-brain axis.

Fasting

When we sleep, we do not eat…indicating a "fast." Fasting is called such because it represents firm will against the temptation of eating food. Waiting to eat until later in the day may prove helpful in the struggle for TBI recovery. Intermittent fasting (IF) involves alternating periods of voluntary fasting or reduced caloric intake with non-fasting, offering adaptable meal timing schedules to promote health and support TBI recovery.[36]

The Importance of Sleep and Sleep Hygiene

TBI sufferers often do not sleep well, and sleep is critical for neural repair and gut health. It is important to understand the

[35] Zou. (May 2025).

[36] See Appendix A for more approaches to IF.

stages of sleep prior to learning how to fix it. Below is a chart with each stage and its characteristics.

Sleep Stage	Characteristics
Stage 1	The lightest stage of sleep occurs as a person first falls asleep
Stage 2	The body relaxes deeply; temperature drops, muscles relax, and heartbeat and breathing slow down
Stage 3	Deep/restorative sleep allows the body to recover and grow
Stage 4	Rapid Eye Movement (REM) sleep; most dreaming occurs, brain activity increases, and the body is temporarily paralyzed

During REM sleep, the brain becomes highly active, resembling wakefulness, while the body remains in a state of temporary paralysis, except for the eyes and breathing muscles. This stage, occurring cyclically every 90 to 120 minutes during sleep, is characterized by vivid dreaming due to heightened neural activity in areas like the amygdala and hippocampus, which process emotions and memories. Heart rate and breathing become irregular, and rapid eye movements occur, likely linked to dream imagery. REM sleep is critical for memory consolidation, emotional regulation, and learning, as it strengthens neural connections formed during the day. REM sleep is crucial for re-learning and healing.

Serotonin, largely gut-derived, and melatonin regulate sleep-wake cycles. The problem with supplementing melatonin is that it is commonly overdosed due to label inaccuracy, and there are mild to moderate side effects. Importantly, if you supplement with serotonin, your body will make less of it. TBIs often disrupt the pathways for melatonin production, leading to insomnia and circadian misalignment.

There are some sleep hygiene practices that will enhance sleep quality and TBI recovery. See the chart below.

Practice	Rationale
Avoid screens 2–3 hours before bedtime	Minimizes blue light exposure
Use blue-blocking glasses in the evening	Preserves melatonin production in the evenings
Avoid bright overhead lights	Switch to low-level soft lights 2 hours before bed
Limit water intake at night	Prevents middle-of-the-night awakenings
Maintain a consistent sleep environment	Helps your body get ready for sleep
Eating meals at least 3 hours before bedtime	To optimize digestion

What worked best for me was to make a "contract" with myself that I would remain in bed without the use of screens, TV, or books for a period of 8 hours per day. This gave me no option to get out of bed except for an occasional trip to the bathroom. I knew I had to remain in bed and would not entertain any other option. This forced me to use the stress and breathing techniques described above, and I wound up falling back asleep.

Mindfulness

Mindful eating is a great practice to reduce gut problems. This equates to eating slowly, expressing gratitude, and checking for satiety. This practice will optimize digestion and nutrient absorption. A gut massage is a gentle self-administered technique of rubbing gently from the lower right side of the abdomen to the top and then across the top and down the left side. Eating until you are about 80% full is also a good guide. Slow down and chew your food, taking a full pause between each bite. Incidentally, I still struggle with this.

Speaking of mindfulness, I wholeheartedly encourage you to take a good look at meditation. There are many resources available for free online. It helps me center myself and figure out how to reduce my stress. One of the most important things we should be doing is figuring out what is truly important and what is just chatter. If we can calm our brain, that will in turn calm our gut and vice versa.

Mindfulness, at its core, is the practice of cultivating intentional awareness of the present moment without judgment. From my perspective, this practice can be viewed as a form of neuroplastic modulation, enabling individuals to rewire neural pathways to enhance emotional regulation and stress resilience.

From my perspective, the interconnectedness of the systems in the body shows the importance of self-regulation as a form of self-care. The human body, or what I colloquially refer to as our "meat suit," is a highly integrated system requiring deliberate maintenance to function optimally. Meditation serves as a non-invasive intervention. This self-work is not selfish; it is a prerequisite for sustained health and productivity. By prioritizing mindfulness, we learn to distinguish between meaningful priorities and the "chatter" of external distractions, a process akin to signal processing in engineering, where noise is filtered to amplify the signal.

For those interested in exploring this further, I recommend seminal texts such as *The Relaxation Response* by Herbert Benson, which explores the physiological benefits of meditation, and *The Mind-Gut Connection* by Emeran Mayer, which delves into the gut-brain axis.[37]

Exercise

Exercise plays a critical role in TBI recovery by enhancing circulation and supporting muscle mass maintenance, both of which contribute to improved physical stability and overall health. For individuals recovering from TBI, regular physical activity boosts blood flow to the brain, delivering essential oxygen and nutrients that aid in neuroplasticity and tissue repair, potentially improving cognitive and motor function. Maintaining muscle mass through targeted exercises, such as resistance training, helps prevent muscle atrophy, which is common during prolonged recovery periods, and enhances stability, reducing the risk of falls, which is a significant concern for TBI patients with impaired balance or coordination. Finally, an important role of exercise is to tire the body physically, making the all-too-important sleep problem more easily overcome.

Exercise should be a daily regimen and include both walking distances longer than 3 miles and weight training. If you need help, seek out a trainer; however, most of this information can be found online. The overall goal is to increase blood flow as well as move the body. Vibration can help drain the glymphatic

[37] See Appendix A for more information on meditation and TBI

system. Vibration or repetitive motion with impact, such as bouncing or jumping, could help remove some of the proteins in the cerebrospinal fluid.

Beyond TBI recovery, preserving muscle mass is vital for human longevity, as it supports metabolic health, bone density, and functional independence. Age-related sarcopenia can lead to frailty and reduced quality of life, but consistent exercise, particularly strength training, mitigates these effects by sustaining muscle strength and endurance, enabling individuals to maintain mobility and vitality well into later years. It should not just be a workout for the sake of working out. This should become part of your life to extend and improve your life. They say move the body, move the bowels, so get in motion to get moving…down there.

Toxin Management

TBI may increase systemic toxin load, as neuroinflammation and gut permeability allow harmful substances to accumulate. Toxins can accumulate in various parts of the body, with some of the most common storage locations being the liver, kidneys, fatty tissues, and blood. Dietary toxins like processed foods, environmental exposures such as pesticides, and stress pollute the body, disrupting the gut microbiome and worsening TBI outcomes.[38] There is also evidence that microplastics are linked to a number of environmental problems and diseases.[39]

Sunlight and Nature

Finally, I emphasize the scientifically validated healing properties of sunlight exposure, which extend beyond mere environmental

[38] See toxins section in Appendix A.

[39] Ririe. (December 2025).

interaction to measurable physiological benefits. Sunlight is a critical source of vitamin D, synthesized in the skin upon UVB exposure, which supports calcium absorption, bone health, and immune function, with studies linking deficiency to increased risks of autoimmune disorders and infections. Morning sunlight, rich in red and near-infrared wavelengths, stimulates serotonin production, enhancing mood and cognitive function by activating pathways in the brain's suprachiasmatic nucleus, which regulates circadian rhythms. Minimizing blue light interference in the evening and integrating red-light exposure promotes melatonin synthesis, thereby improving sleep quality, which is an essential factor for tissue repair and mental health. When I lived underwater for 100 days, I could not obtain vitamin D naturally from the underwater environment. Vitamin D is so important that during that time, 200 IU of vitamin D was the only supplement I took.

Being outdoors amplifies these benefits, as fresh air enhances oxygenation and reduces stress markers such as cortisol. Physical activity during outdoor activities boosts circulation and muscle engagement (see importance discussed above), synergistically supporting cardiovascular health and neuroplasticity. Together, these elements underscore sunlight's role as a multifaceted therapeutic tool, optimizing both immediate well-being and long-term health outcomes.

Stress

I would like to take a moment to talk about physical, psychological, and physiological stress. It is important to stress your body both physically and physiologically. Ten thousand years ago, our ancestors were chased by saber-toothed tigers. That necessitated a healthy, hearty immune system that could respond with things like dopamine, adrenaline, anti-inflammatories, as well as perceptual narrowing to focus on the task at hand… like getting away. This helps by turning off other processes and letting the body focus. That leaves humans with an exceptionally capable and adaptive system which is underutilized today. The biggest stressors are not food, clothing, shelter, or basic survival but something more like the perceived stress of someone not liking something we did online. We can train our system effectively by stressing it minimally which turns out to be a healthy stress. Heathy stressors are the premise behind a process known as hormesis or hormetic response.

For instance, to improve muscle size, we use strength training, which stresses the muscle. When we stress a muscle, we tear the muscle fibers, and the body heals them, making the muscle bigger. That is the same for your entire system and is called hormesis. When you stress your body a little bit in good ways, it can be beneficial to you overall. It can enhance your adaptability and your ability to compensate.

I understand that I just spent a couple of chapters discussing why you should reduce your stress, but we are not talking about the same kind of stress. When you go to the gym and work hard, you put yourself under physical stress, and that is important. When you perform complex mathematical equations, you stress yourself mentally, and that is very important. We are talking about a beneficial kind of stress called hormesis. When your body goes into hormesis, it induces a low level of stress on the cells, triggering an adaptive response that stimulates a repair mechanism. This response and repair will improve overall protection against further stress. Too much stress will wind up hurting you. High levels of stress in the cell can lead to cell damage and apoptosis, or cell death.

You want to focus on things like hormetic levels, which represent the proper level of stress, so the body is challenged but not overly fatigued. This must be accomplished physically, physiologically, and psychologically to improve. This type of hormetic stress can trigger a cascade of cellular processes to enhance overall health, slow aging, and make you more resilient for future stress. It sounds weird, but it is a balancing act.

You can put the body into hormesis by exposure to cold therapy. A caloric deficit also allows your body to induce hormesis.

High stress levels are unsustainable. As your stress levels go up, your cortisol levels rise, and if you are continually there, you are in fight-or-flight. TBI sufferers commonly sit in fight or flight, so it is important to understand that this kind of stress is not good, but cycling stress on and off at moderate levels can be helpful and even prophylactic.

In summary, during recovery you should target the gut-brain axis through synergistic interventions. That means the whole is greater than the sum of its parts. Make attempts to work a combination of the following therapeutic modalities below for best results:

- Diet: Prioritize whole foods, fiber, and fermented products. Explore anti-inflammatory, Mediterranean, or ketogenic diets based on individual needs.
- Exercise: Engage in moderate, preferably outdoor, exercise to enhance gut and brain health.
- Stress Management: Incorporate meditation, breathing exercises, and mindfulness. Relax and remember

mindful eating. Practice intentional, slow eating to optimize digestion and reduce stress.

- Sleep: Adopt rigorous sleep hygiene to support neurotransmitter production.
- Toxin Management: Consider using hyperbaric oxygen therapy (HBOT) under medical guidance. Personalized care is critical, as genetic, metabolic, and cultural factors shape responses. Regular consultation with healthcare providers ensures safety and efficacy.
- Sunlight exposure: Get into the sun. Push for moderate exposures in the early morning and late afternoon if you are fair-skinned.

One major thing of which I am continually reminded is that the human body thrives in changing situations. "Variety is the spice of life." Cycle hormetic stressors to improve your body's ability to cope with stress. Change up whatever food you do and how and when you eat for Constant and Never-Ending Improvement (CANEI). Regardless of how you approach this, whatever menu you choose should be things look forward to eating. Importantly, eat foods that you enjoy and that have flavor. Fad diets do not work, and have been shown to be bad for you. Do not diet; just choose the new way you eat and make it something you can live with. The gut-brain axis is a pivotal determinant of TBI recovery, influencing inflammation, mood, and cognition. By integrating dietary, lifestyle, and integrative strategies, individuals can restore gut health, mitigate neuroinflammation, and enhance resilience. While differences remain in standardizing interventions, a focus on whole foods, mindful living, and individualized care offers a promising framework for optimizing outcomes in TBI survivors. Strategic shopping and toxin avoidance empower patients to heal rapidly, offering a promising framework for TBI management.

Remember, your body wants to heal itself. Prepare and nurture your body to energize it and give it the best support to help it heal itself.

CHAPTER SIX

Blinded by the Need: relationships and brain injury.

"Do you need more discipline ... or a better system?"

BLUF – Your TBI will irrevocably change you. It is important to understand the person who you were may never come back, and the people around you may or may not be able to cope with that. Be kind to yourself and others.

Here is my story in a nutshell: after my TBI, I broke up with a fiancé, Denise; went on a bender in Mexico looking for alternative treatments; and, contemplated suicide before a brave friend (Travis) finally stepped in to help. Travis got me a doctor to help me sleep and he encouraged me. He held me to the standard of the living. His support, combined with what little faith in God I had left and the haunting feeling that I wanted to still be here for my three daughters, allowed me to push past what I had been through. I went through a lot to discover one fundamental truth: a broken brain leads to broken relationships and a broken sense of self.

This chapter gives some advice for people who have a loved one with a traumatic brain injury because I understand first-hand how TBI can change your behavior and your relationships.

The severity of the injury and subsequent changes are hard for both caregiver and patient to understand. From crying in the shower, to facing a drill in my skull while alone in the ICU, to writing a note to my loved one explaining my new needs, I was despondent. I lacked the capacity to reach out for help; it just was not in my makeup. I am usually the person fixing other people's problems.

WARNING

My name is Joe and I have a traumatic brain injury. I may be full of senseless accusations and prone to anger and emotion. The way you treat me is to... be understanding and empathetic and to give me a safe place.

I may be prone to:

Anger / outbursts
Unreasonable emotion
Unbalance or walking disturbances
Suspicion and unreasonable accusations of paranoia
Unreasonable fear / risk taking behavior

What to do and how to handle me

1) Be kind if you love me...just be nice otherwise
2) Work through the paranoia, fear, doubt or emotion with me and DO NOT personalize it
3) Work through the logic and kindly show me where I am wrong
4) Do not yell
5) Do not get angry with me....That has the opposite impact
6) Show me how what I am doing to you is impacting you

How long will this last

Most (80%) TBI / PTSD is correctable in between 3 and 4 months following the incident (if not further provoked)

What can you do to help

Make sure I am sleeping and getting diet and exercise

Denise and I hadn't been together very long when I got into my accident. She was a self-made 30-something woman who had immigrated to the United States from another country. On top of that, she was a beautiful woman with a fitness-model-type body. She was no stranger to hard work, and she devoted her time, effort, and energy to her business. I was in the ICU for two days and the hospital for an additional 5 days. She was only able to visit twice. This highlighted for me her priorities and nature.

Denise noticed the changes in my behavior, and she was struggling to work with this different version of me. I wrote her a sign explaining what I was going through and what she should expect from my TBI. I asked her to be understanding and to give me a safe place. I also reminded her to take care of herself as I recovered. We were at odds, and this was a last-ditch attempt at "righting the ship" when it came to the way that we were interacting. I was trying to help her understand what was wrong with me. This was problematic, to say the least, because she was not very trusting of me at this point, given my erratic behavior.

Behavioral Awareness Checklist

- ☐ **Emotional Volatility**: Overwhelming emotions, such as crying at the drop of a hat or feeling overly emotional and tearing up at the slightest provocation.
- ☐ **Uncontrollable Rage**: Explosive, uncontrollable rage, often directed inward. This includes intense anger at oneself for losing control or not being the man one used to be.
- ☐ **Risk-Taking Behaviors**: Engaging in dangerous activities without concern for safety, such as riding a motorcycle without a helmet, often stemming from a feeling of despondency.
- ☐ **Self-Image/Self-Loathing**: Battling with a residual self-image and hating the person one has become due to cognitive deficits, such as the inability to keep track of basic items like car keys.
- ☐ **Suspicion/Paranoia**: A nagging paranoia or tendency to question the motives of others, even trusted professionals and close associates, assuming they may be cheating or scamming you.

The symptoms of a prefrontal cortex traumatic brain injury are well-documented, and I was a textbook case. First, there are the overwhelming emotions; I was crying at the drop of a hat. Then, there was the anger. Not the kind of anger that simmers quietly, but an explosive, uncontrollable rage. Rage at yourself, mostly. Third, there is risk-taking behavior. And finally, there's suspicion, a nagging paranoia that everyone around you is cheating you in some way. I ticked every box.

I was overly emotional, tearing up at the slightest provocation. At the same time, I was consumed by anger, a fire that burned too hot to contain. I vividly remember gripping the steering wheel of my truck after someone cut me off in traffic, convinced I could rip it clean off and use it as a weapon. When the rage subsided, I would turn that anger inward. I would hate myself for losing control, for not being the man I used to be, and that self-loathing would spiral into massive depression. I had what is referred to as "residual self-image" in the movie "The Matrix;" I had an image of the way I used to be, and I could not live up to it.

And then, there were the risky behaviors. For example, I started riding my motorcycle without a helmet. I told someone, "Well, you got to die of something, so it may as well be this." But it was not bravery or defiance. It was a death wish, plain and simple. I did not want to live like this anymore. I just wanted the pain to stop.

The hardest part was not the physical pain or even the emotional outbursts. It was hating the person I had become. I used to be sharp and capable. I used to remember things. Now? I could not even keep track of my car keys. Not once, not twice, but three times I lost entire sets of keys, forcing me to reorder replacements for my car. Each time felt like another reminder that I was not the same person anymore.

The final symptom that haunted me was suspicion. I began questioning everyone's motives and assuming the worst, even from those I trusted the most. For example, my accountant, Amy, a trusted professional who has had access to every password and handles every dime I spend, suddenly became a source of paranoia. In my mind, she could have been siphoning off money, and I would never know.

One evening, Amy invited me to dinner, as she always did annually, to discuss plans for the next year. During the conversation, she mentioned she had not been paid in three months. Instead of responding rationally, I immediately became suspicious. I thought she was trying to scam me, and I called her on it. I went home, checked my records, and realized the truth… I had not paid her. It was my mistake. I apologized profusely and corrected the issue immediately. The shame from that moment lingered, but it was a stark example of how a TBI warps your ability to trust, even when you have no reason to doubt someone.

Then there was the emotional flood. The amygdala, a small almond-shaped structure deep in the brain that processes emotions, motivation, and behavior, seemed to short-circuit. My emotions overwhelmed me, leaving me unable to manage or even comprehend them. Crying became my new normal. I would sit in the house, lacking any motivation, tears streaming down my face, unable to pinpoint why I was so overwhelmed. It was not a single event or feeling; it was everything, all at once, with no outlet.

For someone like me, who spent decades as a doer in the military, solving problems under pressure and thriving in chaos, this was devastating. Top-level performers, whether in sports, service organizations, or high-stakes professions, thrive on their ability to solve problems and help others. Our sense of purpose is rooted in action, in fixing what is broken. Being told to step aside, to let others take care of you, is a death sentence for people like us.

This is why TBIs hit high performers so hard. We are not just battling physical damage; we are fighting an existential crisis. When you are used to being the person others rely on, losing that ability feels like losing your identity. It is no wonder so many "operator" personalities struggle to cope with TBIs. The idea of being helpless or even worse, a burden, is unbearable. People like me see ourselves as part of the solution, but in this state of mind, we start to see ourselves as part of the problem.

This realization has shaped the way I approach treating TBIs. It is not just about repairing the brain. It is about understanding the person behind the injury… their personality, their purpose, and their identity. Fixing a brain is one thing, but helping someone reclaim their sense of self is another challenge entirely.

I am no saint. Ask anyone who has ever spent an appreciable amount of time with me. This situation was incredibly difficult to deal with for both my fiancé and myself. We had only been together for 9 months, and I had proposed right after my accident. I had ordered the ring before my TBI, so I thought still proposing was the right thing to do. But our relationship was complicated. Besides her business, she was also focused on her nine-year-old child. Importantly, she spent every other weekend with him, which meant she would not be spending that time with me. After the proposal, this became a problem because my unstated expectation was that we would integrate as a family. Integration was not in her plan.

When I asked her to marry me, she was hesitant at first, but then she loved the ring, and she loved being engaged. Shortly thereafter, she realized she lacked the capacity to deal with the situation at hand. The main problem was that she fell in love with somebody and then that person changed.

I admit that I lacked the ability to work with her on our relationship, and my shortcomings contributed to its demise, but one of the reasons why the TBI was the best thing that ever happened to me was because we chose not to get married. We parted about four months after my accident. That turned out to be a wonderful thing in my life because we were not right for each other.

This young lady kept her eyes on her business, not on a relationship with me. Again, that is why I am thankful that it worked out the way it did. In my later years, I have concluded that everything always works out exactly as it is supposed to. Ultimately, my TBI was the best thing that ever happened to me because it meant that I didn't marry someone who wasn't right for me. And yes, I got the diamond back.

When you are dealing with a loved one who has a TBI, and likely in all relationships, a healthy dose of empathy, forgiveness, and love go a long way. It is important to know that I owned my shitty behavior and never (well, truthfully...seldom) used my TBI as an excuse for bad behavior. Ultimately, our attitude is a choice, and we must behave appropriately. Constant change is the new normal with which we now must live. Most importantly, your loved one will face changes which are new and may be permanent. Your relationship may be able to stand these changes. Mine could not. Be kind to each other either way. Empathy is important. Weigh all the facts and the situation as a whole prior to making any rash decisions.

CTE in Sports

Up to this point, we have discussed my experience with TBI, including behavioral changes and other issues I faced during recovery. I have also explained my experience with treating former and current military servicepeople with TBI. However, during the research for this book, I came across additional information on chronic traumatic encephalopathy (CTE) and concussion. A football player's chronic traumatic encephalopathy appears to be a repeated traumatic brain injury. We also see CTE (to a lesser extent) in soccer players.

CTE is associated with neural behavioral dysregulation, particularly in the early stages. Here is how CTE manifests:

- violent, impulsive, or explosive behavior
- aggression and rage
- lack of Behavioral control

CTE in football players is a growing epidemic as well. A 2023 study from Boston University noted that of the autopsies performed on the brains of 376 deceased NFL players, 91.7% of them showed Chronic Traumatic Encephalopathy (CTE).[40] Similar studies found that between 35 and 55% of all players have CTE. Additionally, a 2024 Harvard Football Players Health Study found that one-third of nearly 2,000 living former NFL players believed they had CTE, with higher rates of reported impulsivity, aggression, and depression compared to those without suspected CTE.[41]

For soccer players, repeatedly heading the ball, player-to-player collisions, and falls or collisions with the ground or goalposts cause head injuries and concussions. Repeatedly heading the ball can cause subconcussive impacts, which may accumulate over time and contribute to neurological issues,

[40] *Boston University Chobanian & Avedisian School of Medicine.* (2023).

[41] Wait. (September 2024).

though the link to CTE is less clear than in football. Concussions are the most common form of TBI in soccer, with studies estimating an incidence rate of 0.4 to 1.7 concussions per 1,000 player-hours in professional play.[42]

This fact is exceptionally relevant to the topic at hand: it doesn't matter how you get your hit in the head. It actually is more about how you can recover from it. All of these lifestyle changes can positively affect the outcome of individuals with TBI, regardless of how the TBI occurred.

TBI and Domestic Violence

Sadly, domestic violence (DV) or intimate partner violence (IPV) is a major yet under-recognized cause of TBI, especially mild traumatic brain injury or concussions. Domestic violence can result in TBI through physical acts such as hitting, shaking, strangulation, or throwing objects. A 2020 brain injury study reported that up to 75% of women in domestic violence shelters reported having suffered at least one TBI.[43] There is growing evidence linking long-term domestic violence to CTE-like brain changes. Many of these brain injuries go undiagnosed and untreated, leading to long-term cognitive, psychological, and neurological problems.

---

[42] Mooney. (September 2020),.

[43] Carter. (April 2025).

CHAPTER SEVEN

How to Heal Others Without Losing Your Soul

"Chicken soup for the soul of the healer"

BLUF – This chapter is about the unexpected gift of empathy that came with my recovery and the lessons I have learned about balancing compassion with self-preservation. It is about a chaotic moment in a hyperbaric oxygen therapy chamber that showed me the "depths" (pun intended) of my new emotional awareness and the tightrope walk of caring deeply without losing myself.

The world as I knew it shattered on that morning in September 2021when a reckless driver, late for work, collided with my truck. My 1947 Chevy crumpled like paper and my brain was battered inside its fragile skull. The TBI did not just steal my balance or scramble my thoughts for a time; it rewired who I was. Before the accident, I was driven, focused, maybe even a little too detached. Empathy was a concept I understood but did not deeply feel. After the TBI, something shifted; the injury cracked open a part of me I did not know existed, flooding me with a raw, almost overwhelming capacity to feel the pain of others.

Months into my recovery, I was working at the Undersea Oxygen Clinic offering hyperbaric oxygen therapy, a treatment that had been a lifeline, easing the fog and fatigue of my TBI. I was still navigating my own symptoms of persistent headaches, emotional volatility, and a newfound sensitivity that made me feel the world's weight more acutely. Working at the clinic with others who were suffering felt like a way to give back, to connect with those who understood the disorienting reality of living with a brain injury.

One afternoon, while sitting in my office, my phone rang. It was my lead technician, Victoria. Her voice, usually calm and steady (she was the coolest cucumber I knew), was now shrill, two octaves higher than normal.

"You need to get to the chamber room now," she said, her words clipped with urgency.

My heart raced. Victoria was a stone-cold divemaster who did not panic, so I knew something was seriously wrong. I dropped everything and sprinted to the chamber room, my mind spinning with worst-case scenarios.

When I flew through the door, the scene was chaos. The patient, a large 26-year-old man with a severe TBI that left him with the intellectual capacity of a seven-year-old, was thrashing and screaming in the chamber. He had ripped the speaker and intercom system clean off the chamber's conical end, leaving the aluminum mount twisted and wires dangling like exposed nerves. The air was thick with the smell of feces. Overwhelmed by a sudden, urgent need he could not articulate in time, he had defecated on the bed.

"I told you I had to shit! You should have gotten me out!" He screamed, his voice raw with frustration.

The chamber was nearing the surface, the six-minute ascent almost complete, but the damage was done. This wasn't just a mess; it was a near-catastrophe. The chamber was pressurized with 100% oxygen, a highly flammable environment where a single spark from those torn wires could have ignited an inferno, engulfing the chamber and potentially the entire building. My stomach churned at the thought, but I pushed it aside, focusing on the immediate crisis.

As the chamber reached surface pressure, the patient's mother was there, trying to calm him. He was still belligerent, half-dressed, and resisting her attempts to clean him up.

"I had to shit! Why didn't you listen?" he shouted, his voice breaking.

His mother's face was a mask of exhaustion and defeat, her hands trembling as she tried to soothe him while wiping down his clothes. I glanced at the chamber. The speaker mount was mangled, wires exposed, and the bed was a mess. The damage was significant, likely costing thousands to repair. I looked back at the mother; her eyes, brimming with tears, met mine.

"How much is that (the repair to the chamber) going to cost?" she asked, her voice barely above a whisper, laced with shame and fear.

It was not just about the money; this was another burden, another failure for which she felt responsible. The weight of her struggle was palpable; she was carrying not just this moment but the last year of caregiving, medical appointments, and the relentless unpredictability of her son's condition.

Before my TBI, I might have defaulted to problem-solving mode, rattling off assurances about insurance or repair costs. But my injury had changed me. The raw empathy it unlocked surged through me, and I felt her pain, exhaustion, guilt, and fear of being judged. I saw myself in her, navigating the uncharted waters of a brain injury, and I saw her son, trapped in a body and mind that betrayed him.

Without a second thought, I stepped forward and wrapped my arms around her. She stiffened for a moment, then collapsed into the hug, sobbing quietly. "The chamber will be fixed," I said softly. "Don't worry about it. You're doing a great job...mom."

That moment was a revelation for me. My TBI had given me the ability to see and feel her struggle as if it were my own. However, my new sense of compassion was a mixed blessing. If I were not careful, the weight of my empathy would drag me under unless I learned to balance it.

The Empath's Burden

In the months following my accident, I found myself absorbing the emotions of everyone around me. A friend's frustration, a stranger's grief, even the quiet sadness of a cashier... these all hit me like a tidal wave. I wanted to help, to fix, to heal. But you cannot save everyone, and feeling the pain of others left me drained, with my own recovery faltering under the strain.

Empathy after TBI can feel like a double-edged sword. On the one hand, developing increased empathy was a profound gift because I gained the ability to connect with others in a way that transcends words. On the other hand, I could become exhausted by the burden of taking on the emotions of the people around me.

The incident in the chamber was a stark reminder of this. I could have been consumed by the chaos that I saw around me (the damaged equipment, the near-disaster, the logistical nightmare), but my empathy drew me to the mother's pain.

While that connection was powerful, it left me emotionally spent. This is the empath's burden, especially if the TBI amplifies our emotional sensitivity. The same injury that damages cognitive functions can heighten emotional awareness, leaving us raw and open to the world's suffering. For caregivers, survivors, or anyone navigating life post-TBI, this heightened empathy can be both a strength and a vulnerability. The instinct to help is powerful, but without boundaries, it can erode your own well-being.

Helping others heal from TBI, whether as a caregiver, volunteer, or fellow survivor, requires a delicate balance. The chamber incident was a turning point for me, not just in understanding empathy but in learning how to channel it constructively without letting it consume me. TBI is a complex injury, often invisible, that can leave both the survivor and their supporters grappling with frustration, grief, and impulsiveness. As someone with a TBI, I felt a deep pull to help others navigate this terrain, but I had to learn how to do so without sacrificing my own recovery or sanity. I worked with a therapist who put me on a path to healing others without losing myself. Again... my TBI is proving to be the best thing that ever happened to me. My recovery taught me important lessons I would never have otherwise learned.

Below are the expanded strategies that have guided me on this path, offering a roadmap for anyone seeking to support TBI healing while protecting their own well-being.

Establish Firm Boundaries with Compassion

Boundaries are not about shutting people out; they are about preserving your capacity to help. Remember, if you are struggling to carry your own "pack," you cannot carry another person's pack. You must first set your own pack aside, heal yourself, and then you can help others more. For all the superstar performers out there...when was the last time you set your "pack" down? We all know we can carry more and do more after we rest. It is OK to take some time for self-care...this is not selfish, but actually increases your capacity to give.

After the chamber incident, I realized I could not take on the emotional weight of every patient or caregiver. I set clear limits: offering support during clinic hours but not carrying their stories home. For example, I would listen to the mother's concerns during her son's sessions, but I avoided engaging in long, draining conversations afterward. This allowed me to stay present without becoming overwhelmed. To set boundaries, communicate them kindly but firmly: "I'm here to support you during our time together, and I'll do everything I can in that space." This respects both their needs and your limits.

Develop Emotional Regulation Tools

TBI can amplify emotional responses, making it hard to disentangle your feelings from someone else's. After the chaos in the chamber, I felt a mix of adrenaline, empathy, and guilt for not anticipating the patient's needs. To manage this, I adopted tools like journaling to process emotions after intense moments. This written account of the incident helped me separate my empathy for the mother from my own stress over the damaged chamber. Other tools, like box breathing (inhaling for four counts, holding for four, exhaling for four, and holding the exhale for four counts), or grounding exercises (naming five things you can see, four things you can touch, etc.), can help you stay centered when emotions run high. These practices create a buffer, allowing you to care deeply without being swept away by the emotions of others.

Cultivate Self-Compassion as a Foundation

Helping others heal starts with healing yourself. My TBI left me with a tendency to feel guilty when I could not solve every problem (like the chamber damage or the mother's distress). I had to learn that I was not failing by prioritizing my own recovery. Self-care is not selfish and means treating yourself with the same kindness you offer others. After the incident, I took time to rest, acknowledging that I'd done my best in a crisis. Practical steps include scheduling downtime, celebrating small wins (like completing a day without a headache), and speaking to yourself as you would a friend: "You're doing enough." These steps strengthen your resilience, enabling you to support others without depletion. Taking time to care for yourself will help you be more empathetic and patient. Remember: Self-care is not selfish.

Build a Support Network for Shared Healing

No one can heal others alone, especially with TBI's emotional toll. After the chamber incident, I leaned on my team of friends and the group that normally surrounds me. These connections reminded me I wasn't alone in navigating empathy's challenges. Find or create a network (whether that be a formal group, a therapist, or trusted friends) where you can share the emotional load. Thank you, Travis. For caregivers, this might mean connecting with others who understand the unique strain of supporting someone with a TBI. These spaces allow you to vent, learn, and recharge. We learned during COVID that social connections are important. Loneliness is extremely problematic for humans, and it is rumored that social connections are more valuable than vitamins for well-being. There is also some anecdotal evidence that people with strong social bonds live longer than those without these bonds. It is not about the number of friends but the quality of those relationships; a single person with whom you can be yourself can help you extend and give purpose to your life.

Channel Empathy into Structured Action

Empathy can feel overwhelming when it's undirected, but channeling it into specific actions gives it purpose. After the chamber incident, I worked with the clinic to improve safety protocols, like clearer communication about patient needs during sessions. This gave my empathy a constructive outlet, reducing my sense of helplessness. For others, this might mean volunteering a set number of hours, advocating for TBI awareness, or helping a single person navigate their recovery. Teaching a caregiver about hyperbaric therapy or sharing resources creates a structured action that allows you to focus your compassion without letting it spiral into emotional overload. Purpose cannot be overstated here. It is our drive, on a daily basis, that helps humans survive.

Recognize and Manage Emotional Transference

TBI survivors and caregivers often experience emotional transference, which occurs when a person absorbs or mirrors someone else's pain. In the chamber, I took on the mother's guilt and fear, feeling responsible for her son's outburst. Recognizing this was occurring helped me to step back. I learned to ask, "Is this my emotion, or am I carrying theirs?" If it is theirs, acknowledge it ("I see your pain, and I'm here"), but gently release it. Visualization techniques, like imagining their emotions as a river flowing past you, can help. This allows you to stay connected without internalizing someone else's struggle. This may sound woo-woo or mystical, but I assure you this method works; the spoken word is more powerful than internal thought. I literally had an out loud discussion with myself about this topic in my office, and doing so helped me work through this process the most!

Prioritize Physical and Mental Recovery

TBI recovery demands energy, and overextending empathy can drain you. After the chamber incident, I noticed my headaches worsened from the stress. I had to recommit to my recovery routine: adequate sleep, hydration, and hyperbaric sessions for myself. For caregivers or supporters, this means maintaining your health too. Regular exercise, a balanced diet, and consistent rest are not selfish; they are essential to sustaining your ability to help. Schedule these as non-negotiables, just as you would a therapy session for someone else.

Educate Yourself About TBI's Impact

READ THIS BOOK cover to cover and research the topics I've covered. Get online. Look around for reliable sources. Understanding TBI's emotional and behavioral effects can help you anticipate challenges without taking them personally. The patient's outburst in the chamber was not about the staff or me. It was his brain injury speaking. Learning about TBI's impact on impulse control and emotional regulation helped me respond with patience rather than frustration. For caregivers, studying TBI's effects can prepare you for unpredictable moments, reducing the emotional toll. Knowledge empowers you to help without feeling blindsided. Can I just say...I am proud of you for reading this book: YOU ARE DOING GREAT!

Reduce Cortisol

Cortisol is the root of all evil. It destroys your blood vessels, your immune system, and your brain. The longest-lived people in the world live longer because they exist in harmony with themselves. Importantly, in the TBI state, there is an internal conflict between you and who you try to appear to be. In Japan, the term **Ikigai** refers to "the reason" why you get up in the morning or your purpose in life; you don't have to be on a huge mission, but you must feel a sense of purpose. What matters is feeling like you're needed and that you're here for a reason. Being at peace with who and what you are is important to your life and recovery.

The Path Forward

My TBI didn't just break me; it rebuilt me. The empathy it awakened has been a gift, allowing me to connect with others in ways I never could before. That moment with the mother in the chamber, amidst the chaos of her son's outburst and the damaged equipment, taught me that sometimes a hug can say more than words ever could. But it also showed me that unchecked empathy can become a burden. The near-catastrophe in the chamber, a spark away from disaster, mirrored the internal risk of letting empathy consume me.

You need to protect and preserve your ability to sleep (see chapter on D.E.S.S.E.R.T.S). Additionally, you cannot know "everything" about the best choices for your TBI sufferer, so remember to be kind to yourself. Caring for someone can be rewarding, and it is important to see the little changes and celebrate the little wins. Read up on the importance of mindfulness and breathing exercises… everyone can benefit from being in the present moment. Do your best to not judge your loved one... push them, but try to radically accept their position and new normal.

Helping others heal from TBI is a noble calling, but it is not without cost. This path requires intention, boundaries, and a commitment to your own well-being. By setting limits, regulating emotions, and channeling empathy into action, you can support others without losing yourself. Healing others starts with healing yourself; this is not out of selfishness, but out of necessity. Only by preserving your own light can you guide others through the darkness of TBI. By doing this, you will not just help your loved one heal, but you will grow into a stronger, more compassionate version of yourself, capable of facing the challenges of this new, empathetic life with resilience and grace.

CHAPTER EIGHT

Psychedelics, Dissociatives and other Drugs and their Potential use for TBI Recovery

"Perfect is the enemy of good enough."

BLUF – A look into the deep, dark, and scary world of drugs used to help TBIs…maybe. This chapter will increase your understanding of how drugs work in the body and, importantly, what they can and cannot accomplish. It is specifically not "dumbed down" to increase your knowledge.

The injuries I sustained during my military career hurt both my brain and physical health. The first time I was blown up was my own fault. Then a skydiving accident proved I was not "invincible and invisible". In this chapter, I walk you down the road to understanding what happens when you feel like your body has abandoned you and you learn you are, in fact, only human. That desperate feeling drove me to try anything that might make me better. While my program had a minor component of pharmaceuticals, drugs were not the central focus. My feeling is drugs can and should be used for brief interventions but not become a necessary long-term part of your life. I wish I had this kind of a chapter to read before I tried anything.

Recent research has explored the therapeutic potential of psychedelic and dissociative drugs, such as MDMA, psilocybin, ibogaine, ayahuasca, magic mushrooms, and ketamine, in promoting recovery from TBI. These substances, many of which are illegal in the United States, are being studied for their ability to enhance neuroplasticity (rewire brain connections), reduce inflammation (calm brain swelling), and alleviate co-occurring psychiatric conditions like post-traumatic stress disorder (PTSD), depression, and anxiety (ease mental health issues that often come with TBI).

Below is a brief breakdown of the drugs I have studied in the context of TBI recovery. I include much more information on the pharmacokinetics, pharmacodynamics, research status, and the drug's relevance to TBI recovery.

A Breakdown of TBI Drugs

Drug / Intervention	TBI Relevance	Legal Status	Risks
MDMA	Improves emotional regulation and connectivity.	Schedule I (Illegal)	May worsen hyperarousal.
Psilocybin / Mushrooms	Promotes neurogenesis; reduces anxiety.	Schedule I (Illegal)	Altered consciousness.
Ibogaine	Reduces PTSD; aids synaptic repair.	Schedule I (Illegal)	Cardiotoxicity requires medical supervision.
Ayahuasca	Anti-inflammatory; aids regulation.	Schedule I (Illegal)	Intense effects; nausea.
Ketamine	Increases neuroplasticity and neural complexity.	Schedule III (Legal/Prescription)	Dissociation-induced distress.
Curcumin	Neuroprotective and anti-inflammatory.	Legal (Supplement)	Minimal.
CBD / THC	Neuroprotective; lower mortality link.	Varies by state.	Possible excitotoxicity (THC).
Minocycline	Reduces neuroinflammation.	Legal (Prescription)	Minimal.
Amantadine	Improves cognitive function and arousal.	Legal (Prescription)	Minimal.
Alcohol	Non-therapeutic; worsens injury.	Legal	Impairs recovery; high risk.
Ozempic (Semaglutide)	Potential GLP-1 neuroprotection.	Legal (Prescription)	Minimal.
LSD	Enhances neuroplasticity.	Schedule I (Illegal)	Prolonged stimulation.
Stellate Ganglion Block (SGB)	Improves PTSD, cognition, and recovery.	Legal (Medical procedure)	Hypotension or toxicity risks.

The following list is an exhaustive list meant to help you understand more about how TBI drugs work on your body. It is meant to elevate your knowledge. Pharmacokinetics describes how the body absorbs, spreads, processes, and gets rid of a drug, while pharmacodynamics describes how the drug affects the body's systems and cells. Pharmacokinetics is the study of drug absorption, distribution, and elimination (metabolism and excretion). Pharmacodynamics is the study of the biochemical and physiological effects of a drug and their mechanisms of action at organ system/subcellular/macro cellular levels (how drugs work chemically and physically on areas of the body, from organs to tiny cell parts). Combining these concepts helps you figure out which TBI treatments might work for you or if you should avoid them. Please be aware of the risks of each drug contained within.

TBI Drugs

1. **MDMA:** Commonly known as ecstasy or Molly, MDMA (3,4-methylenedioxyamphetamine) is a synthetic empathogen (man-made drug) that boosts emotional connection by enhancing serotonin, dopamine, and norepinephrine release (AKA the "feel-good" brain chemicals). It is being investigated for its ability to reduce fear and enhance emotional processing without fear, which can be particularly beneficial for veterans with TBI and co-occurring PTSD.[44] Studies suggest MDMA promotes neuroplasticity (forming new brain connections), potentially aiding in rewiring neural

[44] Young. (September 2015)last.

circuits damaged by TBI.[45] A 2017 FDA designation as a breakthrough therapy for PTSD has spurred research, with phase 3 trials showing significant reductions in PTSD symptoms, which often exacerbate TBI-related impairments.[46]

- Pharmacokinetics: MDMA is orally active, with peak plasma concentrations reached in 1.5 to 3 hours. It has a half-life (the amount of time it takes half the consumed drug to leave your body) of 7 to 9 hours, metabolized primarily by the liver via CYP2D6 enzymes into MDA (3,4-methylenedioxy-amphetamine) (broken down by liver enzymes into a related compound). Effects last 3 to 6 hours. Its lipophilic nature allows it to cross the blood-brain barrier (BBB) easily (meaning, it slips into the brain easily due to its fat-friendly structure). Prolonged wakefulness can occur due to its stimulatory effects, often persisting 12 to 24 hours post-dose.
- Pharmacodynamics: MDMA increases serotonin, dopamine, and norepinephrine release by reversing monoamine transporters; in other words, it flips brain chemical switches to release more happy signals. It also acts as a partial agonist at 5-HT2A, 5-HT1A, and 5-HT2C receptors, which enhances emotional processing and reduces fear, beneficial for TBI-related PTSD. MDMA promotes neuroplasticity by increasing BDNF (brain-derived neurotrophic factor, a protein for brain growth),

[45] Peled-Avron. (November 2025).
[46] Feduccia. (September 2019).

potentially aiding neural repair in TBI. Its sympathomimetic effects (e.g., increased heart rate, revs up the body like adrenaline, etc.) may exacerbate hyperarousal in TBI patients, worsening agitation or alertness issues.

- TBI Relevance: Enhances corticolimbic connectivity (strengthens links between thinking and emotion areas of the brain); reduces amygdala hyperactivity (calms the brain's fear center); and supports emotional regulation (helps control moods), addressing TBI-related mood and cognitive deficits. Current research, Phase 3 trials conducted by MAPS (Multidisciplinary Association for Psychadelic Studies) show efficacy for treatment of PTSD, with ongoing studies for treatment of TBI.[47]

2. **Psilocybin and Magic Mushrooms:** Psilocybin, the active compound in magic mushrooms, is a classic psychedelic that acts as a 5-HT2A receptor agonist (triggers a specific serotonin receptor). Upon ingestion, it is converted to psilocin, which crosses the BBB to produce heightened perception, altered consciousness, and increased neuroplasticity (meaning it slips into the brain, changing perception and rewiring connections). Research, including studies from Johns Hopkins, indicates psilocybin can reduce the depression and anxiety common in TBI patients, and promote neurogenesis and synaptogenesis (the growth of new neurons and connections), potentially aiding brain repair.[48] A

[47] A Multi-Site Phase 3 Study of MDMA-Assisted Therapy for PTSD. (December 2023).
[48] Gukasyan. (February 2022).

2025 study highlighted psilocybin's anti-inflammatory properties (reducing brain swelling) and its ability to increase brain network integration (improving brain region teamwork), which may restore cognitive flexibility in TBI patients (helping the brain think in a more flexible way).[49]

- <u>Pharmacokinetics:</u> Psilocybin is orally administered (taken by mouth), and is rapidly dephosphorylated to psilocin in the gut and liver. It peaks in plasma within 1 to 2 hours, with a half-life of 3 hours. Effects last 4 to 6 hours, with residual stimulation potentially causing wakefulness for 8 to 12 hours (it may keep you awake after taking it). Psilocin crosses the BBB efficiently.
- <u>Pharmacodynamics:</u> Psilocin: alters perception and increases neural plasticity (changes how you see and think, boosting brain flexibility); enhances BDNF and synaptogenesis (grows neurons and connections); reduces neuroinflammation (calms brain swelling); and increases brain network integration, as shown in 2025 Johns Hopkins studies.[50] These effects may restore cognitive flexibility in patients with TBI.
- <u>TBI Relevance:</u> Anti-inflammatory properties and enhanced neurogenesis may aid repair of TBI-damaged neural circuits, and may be effective for depression and anxiety, which are common with TBI.

[49] Koseli. (May 2025).
[50] Davis. (November 2025).

3. **Ibogaine:** Ibogaine is a psychoactive indole alkaloid derived from the root bark of the Tabernanthe iboga shrub or the Voacanga Africana plant, native to Gabon in West Africa. Traditionally used in Bwiti spiritual practices, ibogaine was described scientifically in 1889. Anecdotal reports from the region note animals (e.g., gorillas) consuming the root during grief, suggesting a possible role in processing trauma. Ibogaine is known for its intense, dream-like effects and its potential for treating addiction, PTSD, and TBI, though it carries significant risks and requires medical supervision.
    - Pharmacokinetics: Ibogaine is typically administered orally. It is rapidly absorbed, with effects onset within 1 to 2 hours. Ibogaine has a half-life of approximately 7 to 8 hours in extensive CYP2D6 metabolizers, while noribogaine has a much longer half-life of 28 to 49 hours (or more), leading to prolonged activity. Individual variability in CYP2D6 genetics strongly affects exposure and clearance. It is lipophilic, crosses the BBB readily, and is eliminated primarily through hepatic metabolism with some renal excretion.
    - Pharmacodynamics: Ibogaine has a complex, multi-target profile: non-competitive antagonist at nicotinic acetylcholine receptors (notably α3β4), which may reduce reward from nicotine and other substances; NMDA (N-methyl-D-aspartate) glutamate receptor antagonist (contributes to anti-addictive and rapid antidepressant effects); and, interactions with opioid (μ and κ), serotonin (including SERT inhibition via noribogaine), sigma-1/2, and

dopamine systems. It promotes neuroplasticity by increasing BDNF and GDNF expression, supporting synaptic repair and rewiring. Noribogaine acts as a serotonin reuptake inhibitor and κ-opioid agonist, contributing to mood stabilization and reduced cravings. These actions can interrupt withdrawal, reset addiction-related circuits, reduce inflammation/excitotoxicity (relevant to TBI), and facilitate profound psychological processing of trauma.

- TBI/PTSD Relevance: In a 2024 prospective observational study, no serious adverse events occurred with magnesium co-administration.[51] Preclinical and other human data support neuroprotection, anti-inflammatory effects, and enhanced plasticity.
- Legal Status: Ibogaine is a Schedule I controlled substance in the United States (high abuse potential, no accepted federal medical use), making it illegal to possess, distribute, or administer outside approved research. However, clinical research is advancing, with FDA IND clearances and state-level interest increasing (e.g., legislative funding in Texas). It is available under medical supervision in Brazil (with prescription use legalized in São Paulo in 2016 and expanding) and certain other countries (e.g., Mexico clinics). Ibogaine is not FDA-approved for any indication. The truth appears to be that its abuse potential is zero, since the experience of taking ibogaine is uncomfortable, in my opinion.

[51] Cherian. (2024).

- Important Cautions and Practical Guidance: This is a powerful substance with real risks, including cardiotoxicity, QT prolongation, and arrhythmias. It must not be undertaken lightly or as "bro science," a term that refers to science based on anecdotal evidence. Medical screening (especially cardiac), ECG monitoring, and magnesium co-administration are essential. Work only with trained professionals. Nausea, vomiting, and dizziness are to be expected.
- Recommended Practitioner: Dr. Bruno Rasmussen Chaves in Brazil has over 30 years of experience as a medical doctor and researcher who is the pioneer in ibogaine treatments in clinical settings, often combined with psychotherapy. Visit him or similarly qualified medical teams.
- Preparation Tips: Consume only a light meal the evening before, and fast on treatment day (nausea and vomiting are common). Use an eye mask for an internal journey. Prepare 4+ hours of instrumental or minimally lyrical music (e.g., Gregorian chants). Emotional releases and vivid visions/hallucinations (visual + auditory) are typical.
- Post-Treatment: Sleep is disrupted for ~72 hours (ibogaine/noribogaine suppress REM). Expect post-acute dizziness/ataxia ("off a boat" sensation). Stay hydrated; avoid massage initially if it worsens motion issues. First 72 hours: Tranquil environment with psychological support. First 30 days: Critical neuroplasticity window. Avoid addictive stimuli (social media, alcohol, nicotine) and build positive

habits. Maintain fitness, red light therapy, contrast therapy, etc.

- Nicotine/caffeine note: Both can reduce BDNF; minimizing them supports recovery.
- Dosing (Experiential/Clinical Guidance): Common ranges: 8 to 12+ mg/kg for addiction/PTSD; test doses of 2 3 mg/kg are often used. Practitioners may vary the dose slightly based on the sex or metabolism of the patient, but evidence for proper dosing is limited.
- Ibogaine shows remarkable promise but demands respect, preparation, and integration. It is not a stand-alone cure. Taking ibogaine in a group dynamic and environment, as typically occurs, may play a large role in efficacy because the post-experience period solidifies new pathways. Prioritize safety with qualified medical professionals and cardiac monitoring.

4. **Ayahuasca:** Ayahuasca, a South American brew containing DMT (N, N-dimethyltryptamine) and β-carboline alkaloids, is a classic psychedelic that enhances neuroplasticity and increases BDNF (boosts brain growth). Ayahuasca may increase serum BDNF levels for 48 hours (supporting growth of neuron branches and connections), which may aid TBI recovery. Its effects last 4 to 8 hours, with DMT's half-life being approximately 15 to 60 minutes when combined with monoamine oxidase inhibitors in ayahuasca. Research is limited, but preliminary data suggest benefits for depression and PTSD, which often complicate TBI recovery.[52]

[52] Khan. (September 2021).

- Pharmacokinetics: Ayahuasca is a brew combining DMT (not orally active alone) with β-carboline alkaloids (harmine, harmaline) that inhibit MAO, allowing DMT absorption. DMT peaks in plasma within 1 to 2 hours, with a half-life of 15 to 60 minutes, while β-carbolines extend effects to 4–8 hours. Excretion is primarily urinary. Prolonged wakefulness (up to 12 hours) may occur due to MAO inhibition and serotonergic stimulation.
- Pharmacodynamics: DMT produces intense psychedelic effects. It enhances serotonin levels and inhibits MAO-A. Ayahuasca increases BDNF and spinogenesis, supporting neural repair. It reduces default mode network (DMN) activity (calms overactive brain patterns), potentially aiding emotional regulation in TBI.
- TBI Relevance: BDNF increase and anti-inflammatory effects may support TBI recovery; benefits for depression and PTSD are relevant for TBI comorbidities.

5. **Ketamine and Dissociatives:** Ketamine, a dissociative anesthetic and NMDA receptor antagonist (blocks a specific brain signal), is a non-classic psychedelic with rapid antidepressant effects. It is legally available as a Schedule III drug in the United States for anesthesia and, since 2019, as esketamine (Spravato) nasal spray for treatment-resistant depression. Studies indicate ketamine increases neural complexity and promotes neuroplasticity (boosts brain flexibility and growth), potentially aiding TBI

recovery by restoring links between thinking and emotion areas. [53] Other dissociatives, like PCP and dextromethorphan (DXM), are less studied for TBI due to higher risks of psychosis and abuse potential. Cognitive Behavioral Therapy (CBT), while not a drug, is a legal, evidence-based treatment for TBI-related psychiatric symptoms, often used alongside ketamine in clinical settings.

- Pharmacokinetics: Ketamine is administered intravenously, intranasally (esketamine), sublingual (troches), or intramuscularly, peaking in plasma within 5 to 30 minutes (IV) or 20 to 40 minutes (intranasal). It has a half-life of 2 to 3 hours. Effects last 1 to 2 hours, but residual alertness may persist for 6 hours due to dissociative properties.
- Pharmacodynamics: As an NMDA receptor antagonist, ketamine disrupts glutamatergic signaling, increasing neural complexity and BDNF. It rapidly reduces depression via mTOR pathway activation and enhances corticolimbic connectivity. Its dissociative effects may help TBI patients process trauma.
- TBI Relevance: Promotes neuroplasticity and alleviates depression, addressing TBI-related cognitive and mood impairments. Esketamine is FDA-approved for depression.
- Legal Status: Schedule III (legal) for anesthesia; esketamine approved for depression.

[53] Zanza. (March 2022).

6. **Nutraceuticals**: Compounds like omega-3 fatty acids, curcumin, and N-acetylcysteine (NAC) are widely available, cost-effective, and may support TBI recovery when combined with other therapies, though evidence is less robust than for psychedelics. **NAC** is an anti-oxidant and anti-inflammatory (fights cell damage and swelling), which may reduce oxidative stress in TBI (calms harmful chemical reactions).
   - Pharmacokinetics: Orally administered, peaks in 1 to 2 hours, half-life of 5.6 hours. Metabolized in the liver, excreted in urine. Well-tolerated with minimal wakefulness effects.
   - Pharmacodynamics: Antioxidant that replenishes glutathione (a protective molecule), reducing oxidative stress and neuroinflammation. May modulate glutamate (balances brain signals), supporting TBI recovery.
   - TBI Relevance: Small studies suggest benefits for mild TBI and neuroprotection.[54]
7. **Curcumin:** This bright yellow phenolic compound is the main constituent of turmeric powder, and used as a food coloring, flavoring, and dietary supplement. It is anti-inflammatory and neuroprotective; it may reduce neuroinflammation post-TBI.
   - Pharmacokinetics: Poor oral bioavailability, peaks in 1 to 2 hours, half-life of 6 to 7 hours. Enhanced with piperine to improve absorption. Excreted via bile.

[54] Lucke. (October 2016).

- Pharmacodynamics: Anti-inflammatory and antioxidant. It blocks harmful immune signals. Preclinical data suggest neuroprotection in TBI.[55]
- TBI Relevance: Preclinical studies appear promising, but there is limited human data for reducing neuroinflammation.

8. **CBD and THC:** CBD, legal in many states, has shown neuroprotective effects in TBI models (protects brain cells).[56] CBD has neuroprotective and anti-inflammatory effects, and THC is linked to reduced TBI mortality.[57]
    - Pharmacokinetics: CBD peaks in 2 to 4 hours (oral), with a half-life of 18 to 32 hours. THC peaks in 1 to 2 hours, with a half-life of 25 to 36 hours. Both are excreted in urine and feces.
    - Pharmacodynamics: CBD modulates CB1/CB2 receptors (adjusts cannabis-related brain signals), reduces inflammation, and has neuroprotective effects. THC activates CB1, reducing excitotoxicity (overactive brain signals). Observational data link THC to lower TBI mortality.
    - TBI Relevance: CBD shows promise in preclinical models; THC needs more study.
9. **Minocycline:** Minocycline is an antibiotic with anti-inflammatory and neuroprotective properties (fights

[55] Guo. (May 2024).
[56] Hergert. (January 2025).
[57] Nguyen. (October 2014).

swelling and protects brain cells); may reduce secondary TBI damage.

- Pharmacokinetics: Orally administered, peaks in 2 to 3 hours, half-life of 11 to 23 hours. Crosses BBB, excreted in urine and feces.
- Pharmacodynamics: Tetracycline antibiotic with anti-inflammatory and anti-apoptotic effects (prevents cell death). Inhibits microglia activation (calms immune cells in the brain), reducing secondary TBI damage.
- TBI Relevance: Phase 2 trials show potential in acute TBI.[58]

10. **Progesterone:** A steroid hormone released by the corpus luteum (hormone from the reproductive system), progesterone may be neuroprotective and reduces edema and inflammation post-TBI (lessens brain swelling).
    - Pharmacokinetics: Administered IV or orally, peaks in 1 to 3 hours, half-life of 16 to 18 hours. Metabolized in the liver, excreted in urine.
    - Pharmacodynamics: Neuroprotective, reduces edema and inflammation. Calms brain signals and immune responses. May promote myelination (rebuilds nerve insulation).
    - TBI Relevance: Trials showed mixed results, with some benefit in acute TBI.[59]

[58] Bergold. (September 2023).
[59] Espinoza. (November 2011).

11. **Amantadine:** Amantadine is a dopamine agonist (boosts dopamine) which may improve cognitive function and arousal in TBI patients (helps thinking and alertness).
    - Pharmacokinetics: Orally administered, peaks in 2 to 4 hours, half-life of 10 to 31 hours. Excreted unchanged in urine.
    - Pharmacodynamics: Dopamine agonist and weak NMDA antagonist, increases dopamine release and arousal. Improves cognitive function in TBI.
    - TBI Relevance: Studies support modest cognitive recovery in moderate to severe TBI.[60]
    - Legal Status: Legal, but prescription-only.
12. **Alcohol:** Alcohol is a psychoactive substance commonly consumed in beverages. It acts as a central nervous system (CNS) depressant (slows brain activity), affecting mood, cognition, and motor function. Some cultures and traditions believe that alcohol has a spiritual connection because it can be used in rituals and ceremonies to connect with the divine or to symbolize transformation and purification. The idea of alcohol as a "spirit" can be seen as both a literal reference to its transformative process and a metaphorical one about its effect on the human spirit or consciousness.
    - Pharmacokinetics: Liquid drink is rapidly absorbed in the stomach and small intestine; peak blood concentrations occur within 30 to 90 minutes

[60] Loggini. (2020),the .

after ingestion. Primarily metabolized in the liver. Excreted mainly in urine breath, and sweat.

- Pharmacodynamics: Acts on GABA-A receptors (enhances inhibition; calms brain), NMDA receptors (inhibits excitation; blocks overactivity), and dopamine pathways (increases reward signaling; boosts feel-good signals). Causes sedation, impaired coordination, and, at high doses, respiratory depression or coma.
- TBI Relevance: Alcohol is not a therapeutic agent for TBI and may exacerbate outcomes (worsen recovery). Studies show acute alcohol intoxication at the time of TBI worsens secondary brain injury, increases mortality, and impairs recovery due to enhanced excitotoxicity and inflammation (overactive brain signals and swelling). Chronic alcohol use pre-TBI is linked to poorer cognitive outcomes.

13. **Body Protection Compound 157:** Known as BPC-157, this compound is a synthetic peptide derived from human gastric juice protein. It is investigated for cytoprotective and healing properties (protects and repairs cells).
    - Pharmacokinetics: Bioavailable via oral, intraperitoneal (IP), intramuscular (IM), or intravenous (IV) routes; stable in gastric juice. Distribution: Rapidly metabolized into small peptide fragments and amino acids; half-life <30 minutes in rats and dogs. Primarily urine and bile excretion.
    - Pharmacodynamics: Promotes tissue repair, angiogenesis (blood vessel growth), and collagen

formation via pathways like FAK-paxillin; modulates inflammation (reduces IL-6, TNF-α; calms immune signals). Counteracts neurotransmitter imbalances (dopamine, serotonin, glutamate, NO systems) and NSAID-induced toxicity.

- TBI Relevance: BPC-157 (10 μg or 10 ng/kg IP) post-TBI (falling weight model) reduced brain edema, hemorrhagic lacerations, and mortality, improving consciousness and outcomes at force impulses of 0.068–0.145 Ns. Prophylactic use (30 min pre-TBI) further lowered unconsciousness and death rates. Studies suggest BPC 157 may serve as a remedy in various CNS-disorders.[61]

14. **Ozempic (Semaglutide):** Ozempic is a brand name for semaglutide, a synthetic GLP-1 receptor agonist (39 amino acids) used for type 2 diabetes, weight management, and in some cases to help with TBIs.
    - Pharmacokinetics: Administered via subcutaneous injection. It is degraded by proteolytic enzymes; not primarily liver-metabolized. Finally, it is eliminated via urine and feces; half-life ~1 week, allowing weekly dosing.
    - Pharmacodynamics: Mimics GLP-1, enhancing insulin secretion, reducing glucagon release, and slowing gastric emptying, leading to glycemic control and appetite suppression (controls blood sugar and reduces hunger). May have neuroprotective effects via GLP-1 receptor activation in the brain.

[61] Sikiric. (2016).

- TBI Relevance: No direct studies on semaglutide for TBI. Preclinical data on GLP-1 agonists (e.g., exenatide) suggest neuroprotection in TBI models by reducing inflammation and apoptosis (cell death).[62] Semaglutide's long half-life and BBB penetration suggest potential, but human TBI trials are lacking. Indirect relevance: TBI patients with diabetes may benefit from semaglutide's glycemic control, potentially reducing secondary injury from hyperglycemia (high blood sugar).

15. **Synapsin:** It refers to a family of endogenous phosphoproteins (Synapsins I, II, III) critical for synaptic vesicle regulation in neurons (controls how neurons release signals). In TBI contexts, synapsin is a synthetic analog or formulation (e.g., nasal sprays combining peptides like Selank) marketed for neuroprotection.

    - Pharmacokinetics: Endogenous synapsins regulate neurotransmitter release by tethering synaptic vesicles to the cytoskeleton (control signal release in neurons); altered in TBI, contributing to synaptic dysfunction (disrupted brain communication). Potentially reduces anxiety and improves cognition. Mechanisms are speculative without robust data.
    - Pharmacodynamics: Endogenous synapsins regulate neurotransmitter release by tethering synaptic vesicles to the cytoskeleton; altered in TBI, contributing to synaptic dysfunction. These claim to modulate GABA, enkephalins, and neurotrophic factors (e.g.,

[62] Harej. (October 2024).

BDNF), potentially reducing anxiety and improving cognition. Mechanisms are speculative without robust data.

- TBI Relevance: No direct therapeutic trials. Synthetic synapsin formulations (e.g., nasal sprays): No peer-reviewed TBI studies. Anecdotal claims suggest neuroprotection or cognitive enhancement, but evidence is lacking. Selank, sometimes included, has preclinical data for anti-anxiety effects but no TBI-specific trials.
- Legal Status: Endogenous synapsins are not drugs; therefore, there is no legal status. Synthetic formulations are not FDA-approved. They are often sold as "research chemicals" or supplements, often with disclaimers. Their legal status is unclear, likely unregulated in many jurisdictions. WADA status unknown but potentially falls under S0 (non-approved substances) if used in sports.

16. **Other Peptides Used in TBI:** Peptides investigated for TBI include Cerebrolysin, Selank, and thymosin beta-4 (TB4), often for neuroprotection or regeneration. Cerebrolysin is the most studied.

    - Pharmacokinetics (General for Peptides, Specifics Vary): Commonly administered IV (Cerebrolysin), IM, or intranasally (Selank, TB4). The bioavailability varies (low oral bioavailability for most peptides). Some peptides, like Cerebrolysin, cross the BBB due to small peptide fragments, while others (e.g., TB4) act peripherally or locally. Metabolism is rapidly degraded by peptidases; half-lives typically range from minutes to hours. Renal clearance of peptide fragments and amino acids.

- Pharmacodynamics: Cerebrolysin is a mixture of neurotrophic peptides which enhances neuronal survival, neurogenesis, and BDNF expression (promotes brain cell survival and growth). Selank potentially aids in cognition (calms stress and may improve thinking). It also promotes cell migration, angiogenesis, as well as anti-inflammatory effects, and may support axonal repair (helps repair nerve fibers).
- TBI Relevance: Cerebrolysin has multiple trials showing efficacy in TBI.[63]
- Legal Status: Cerebrolysin is approved in some countries (e.g., Europe, Asia) for TBI and stroke; not FDA-approved in the U.S. Prescription-only where approved. Selank is not FDA-approved and is sold as a research chemical in some regions. WADA bans it under S0 (non-approved substances). Thymosin Beta-4 is not FDA-approved and would be for investigational use only. WADA-banned under S0.

17. **Other Psychedelics:** LSD and 5-MeO-DMT are under investigation for their neuroplasticity-enhancing effects (brain rewiring). LSD, a 5-HT2A receptor agonist, has shown promise in increasing brain complexity, similar to psilocybin, but lacks extensive TBI-specific research. 5-MeO-DMT, found in certain toads and

[63] Jarosz. (March 2023).

plants, has been anecdotally linked to PTSD symptom relief in veterans. LSD, with a half-life of 3 to 5 hours and effects lasting 8–12 hours (LSD), and 5-MeO-DMT, with a half-life of 15–30 minutes and effects lasting 1–2 hours, can cause prolonged wakefulness due to their stimulatory effects on the central nervous system. They are both Schedule I substances (meaning, illegal) with minimal TBI research.

18. **Stellate Ganglion Block** (SGB): SGB is a medical procedure involving the injection of a local anesthetic, such as bupivacaine, into the stellate ganglion (a cluster of nerves in the neck) to temporarily interrupt sympathetic nervous system signals. This block has been investigated for its potential in managing symptoms associated with TBI, including PTSD-like symptoms, pain, dysphagia (swallowing difficulties), and neurobehavioral issues. Research suggests SGB may modulate brain hemodynamics, reduce intracranial pressure, and improve overall recovery by alleviating inflammation and sympathetic overactivity. While not a drug itself, the procedure relies on anesthetics like bupivacaine or ropivacaine, and some studies indicate benefits for veterans and TBI patients.[64] Evidence is emerging and requires further validation.

    - Pharmacokinetics: For bupivacaine (a commonly used anesthetic in SGB), systemic absorption is dependent on the dose, concentration, route of administration, vascularity of the site, and presence

[64] Lipov. (2023).

of epinephrine. It has a half-life of approximately 2.7 hours in adults (longer in neonates at 8.1 hours), with extended formulations reaching 15 to 17 hours.

- Pharmacodynamics: Bupivacaine is an amide local anesthetic that blocks the generation and conduction of nerve impulses by inhibiting voltage-gated sodium channels on the intracellular side of nerve membranes, stabilizing the membrane and preventing depolarization. This results in a use-dependent block, more pronounced during repetitive activity. Additionally, it may bind to prostaglandin E2 receptors (EP1 subtype), inhibiting prostaglandin production and contributing to anti-inflammatory and analgesic effects. At therapeutic doses, effects on cardiac conduction and peripheral resistance are minimal, but toxic levels can cause CNS stimulation/depression, cardiac arrhythmias, and vasodilation leading to hypotension.
- TBI Relevance: SGB has shown promise in TBI by modulating cerebral hemodynamics, lowering intracranial pressure, and providing neuroprotection. Clinical trials indicate improvements in disability, PTSD, depression, cognition, dysphagia, and activities of daily living, particularly in veterans with mild TBI.[65] It may also reduce secondary brain injury by inhibiting inflammation and endothelial dysfunction.

[65] Mulvaney. (November 2024).

- Legal Status: SGB is a legal medical procedure in the United States when performed by qualified healthcare professionals. The anesthetics used, such as bupivacaine, are FDA-approved for local and regional anesthesia. It requires a prescription and is typically administered in clinical settings; it is not specifically scheduled as a controlled substance but is subject to medical regulations.

The Veterans Health Administration is funding trials for MDMA and psilocybin to treat PTSD and depression in veterans, reflecting growing interest in psychedelic-assisted therapy.[66] However, challenges include the difficulty of conducting double-blind trials due to psychedelics' strong psychoactive effects and ethical concerns about administering these drugs to vulnerable populations, such as those with disorders of consciousness (impaired awareness).

In the chapter on D.E.S.S.E.R.T.S you'll learn that TBI sufferers have difficulty sleeping. Some of these drugs' stimulatory or dissociative properties can disrupt sleep, as found in therapeutic settings where patients are monitored post-administration. Therefore, using these drugs requires careful management to avoid fatigue or exacerbation of TBI symptoms (worsening TBI issues).

Stellate Ganglion Block (SGB) has shown particularly good results in helping symptoms of TBI and PTSD when performed in combination with therapy. Again, the combination of treatment modalities helps in almost every aspect. While psychedelics and dissociatives show promise for TBI recovery,

[66] *U.S. Department of Veterans Affairs.* (December 2024).

significant hurdles remain. The risk of adverse effects, such as ibogaine's cardiac toxicity or ketamine's potential for dissociation-induced distress, necessitates careful medical supervision. The placebo effect in microdosing studies, and the difficulty of blinding trials due to psychoactive effects, complicate research. Ethical concerns, particularly around consent in patients with severe TBI or disorders of consciousness, also pose challenges.

This is by no means an all-inclusive list of every drug used in TBI recovery, but it does highlight some of the more prevalent ones. I believe that future drug research should focus on larger, randomized controlled trials to confirm efficacy and safety. Additionally, research could benefit from the development of non-hallucinogenic analogs (e.g., ibogaine derivatives) to reduce psychological risks. As seems evident, psychedelics should be combined with psychotherapy and nutraceuticals to enhance outcomes. In the long term, I envision policy changes to facilitate research.

Overall, there is potential to address TBI's complex pathology through neuroplasticity, anti-inflammatory effects, and psychiatric symptom relief. MDMA, psilocybin, ibogaine, ayahuasca, and ketamine show promise but are largely illegal, with ongoing research exploring their efficacy. Legal alternatives like NAC, omega-3s, curcumin, minocycline, progesterone, and amantadine offer varying degrees of neuroprotection and symptom relief, though evidence is less robust. Careful consideration of the effects on wakefulness and legal barriers is essential for integrating these compounds into TBI treatment protocols. While most are illegal in the United States, ongoing research, particularly at institutions such as Stanford and Johns Hopkins, is building a case for their therapeutic potential. Ketamine and nutraceuticals provide legal alternatives, but their efficacy for TBI-specific outcomes requires further study. As research progresses, these compounds may revolutionize TBI treatment, offering hope to veterans and others with persistent neurological impairments. I believe you should research any drug you put in your body and not just relying on "bro science". Bro science is doing whatever your "bro" did. Remember, there are consequences for everything you put in your body.

CHAPTER NINE

Project NEPTUNE 100 – and the Next Chapter

"Science is the understanding of the behavior of nature."

- Richard Feynman

BLUF – This chapter reflects on a project in which I use biomedical engineering to illustrate the mechanisms of hyperbaric medicine while advancing STEM education and ocean conservation. It highlights the Brain Optimization Lab and similar centers that push the boundaries of TBI recovery by safely stacking modalities such as HBOT, neurofeedback, and other treatments, tailored to individual needs and guided by evidence-based safety protocols.

As I sat there in the Jules Undersea Lab, 22 feet underwater, living in a unique habitat, I found myself reflecting on the past year and a half. It is no coincidence that I was at nearly the same depth and pressure where I discovered hyperbaric medicine as a treatment for traumatic brain injury. In life, I opine it is best to aim for as many targets as possible with a single arrow, and Project NEPTUNE 100, my mission at the Jules Undersea Lab, did exactly that. This 100 day undersea living experiment was multifaceted, with goals that included but were not limited to:

1. Conducting research on the human body in an isolated, confined, and extreme environment. The aim was to better understand how the body adapts to hyperbaric pressure and to gather data relevant to long-duration spaceflight, such as a 200-day journey to Mars.
2. Educating students about marine environments and inspiring careers in science, technology, engineering, and math (STEM). We had direct contact with over 5,500 students in 19 different countries.
3. Hosting world-renowned experts in fields like shark physiology, benthic geology, marine science, microbiology, sponges, and hyperbaric medicine. Together, we shared knowledge about preserving, protecting, and rejuvenating our marine environment. Approximately 50% of Earth's oxygen comes from the ocean, making its protection a critical priority.[67] We were also working to educate the next generation on safeguarding this vital resource.
4. Raising awareness about treatments for TBI and post-traumatic stress disorder (PTSD) using hyperbaric medicine. My mission also highlighted the mechanisms of action behind hyperbaric treatments and sheds light on alternative methods for healing the brain. By helping the general population understand how these therapies work, my hope was that they would see the

[67] "How Much Oxygen Comes from the Ocean?" NOAA's National Ocean Service. Accessed June 5, 2026. https://oceanservice.noaa.gov/facts/ocean-oxygen.html.

> potential to apply them not just to TBI and PTSD, but to a wide range of conditions, allowing natural healing to take place in the human body.

On May 16, 2023, I broke the previous world record (73 days) for the most time living underwater (at sea pressure) during this Project NEPTUNE 100 mission at the Jules Undersea Lab in Key Largo, Florida. It's no coincidence I chose to live 100 days at the same depth and under the same pressure used to cure my own TBI. The mission gained international attention and has allowed me to share my story of TBI and new TBI protocols; it has also enabled me to invite environmental experts into my undersea habitat and conduct 200 interviews with media around the world. When I came out of the water the day after World Ocean Day (June 9, 2023), I shared myriad details from my 100 days in the approximately 100-square-foot habitat.

This underwater odyssey was not just a stunt or a record-breaking endeavor; it was a profound extension of my TBI recovery journey. Emerging from that habitat, I felt not only physically rejuvenated but intellectually charged to push the boundaries of what we know about brain healing.

The Next Steps in TBI Recovery

My time below the surface reinforced a key lesson: true recovery often comes from stacking modalities or combining therapies in innovative, safe ways to amplify their effects. It is about treating the brain as a dynamic system, not a broken machine that can be fixed with a single tool. TBI sufferers need treatment that focuses on the whole person and gives them hope for the future.

This chapter explores the "next steps" in TBI recovery, spotlighting cutting-edge labs and centers that embody this philosophy. These labs are where science meets resilience, paving the way for anyone grappling with the aftermath of a brain injury.

At the forefront of this movement is the Brain Optimization Lab (BOL). BOL specializes in addressing catastrophic injuries like TBI and CTE through a multidisciplinary approach, but its focus is on optimization, not treatment per se. We are not just talking about traditional rehab; we are talking about optimizing the brain's potential by integrating advanced diagnostics, personalized protocols, and stacked therapies. Stacking modalities means combining therapies that complement each other.

For example, at BOL, they may combine the following therapies:

- HBOT to oxygenate tissues
- neurofeedback to retrain patterns
- psychedelics (always under clinical supervision) for neuroplasticity
- nutraceuticals for anti-inflammatory support and cellular repair

The lab's work on TBI rehabilitation emphasizes safety first: every modality is evidence-based, monitored by experts, and tailored to the individual's biomarkers and symptoms. The key is supervision: qualified professionals monitor interactions, adjust dosages, and use biomarkers (such as blood tests or EEGs) to ensure safety. This is not do-it-yourself experimentation; it is precision medicine.

At BOL, a patient might undergo HBOT sessions to boost oxygen delivery, followed by transcranial magnetic stimulation (TMS) to stimulate dormant brain areas, all while incorporating mindfulness or biofeedback to manage stress responses.

What makes BOL stand out is its commitment to pushing boundaries without recklessness. I am working with them, and we collaborate with neuroscientists, biomedical engineers, and clinicians to "stack" modalities by layering them synergistically. This is not experimental guessing; it is grounded in data from ongoing studies showing how these combinations can accelerate recovery, reduce chronic symptoms like headaches and fatigue, and even prevent secondary complications like depression. If you are a veteran, athlete, or accident survivor dealing with TBI, places like BOL offer hope beyond standard care; they treat you as a whole person, not just a diagnosis.

The Brain Optimization Lab is not alone in this revolution. Across the country and beyond, similar centers are redefining TBI treatment by safely stacking modalities to achieve breakthroughs. The result? Anecdotally, individuals have significant improvements in focus, memory, and emotional regulation. These individuals report 75% symptom reduction in post-concussion syndrome cases. It's safe, non-invasive, and backed by peer-reviewed research, making it a beacon for those frustrated with conventional neurology.

Other treatment protocols use scans to visualize brain activity, then stack interventions like targeted supplements (e.g., omega-3s for inflammation), HBOT, and neurofeedback. TBI patients often receive TMS or low-level laser therapy to promote cellular healing. What I appreciate about all these new treatment places is their emphasis on personalization. No two brains are alike, so no two stacks are identical.

This approach has helped thousands, including veterans with comorbid PTSD, by addressing the root causes rather than just symptoms.

There is a lab in Atlanta, Georgia, that focuses on mild TBI in civilians, veterans, and first responders. They stack modalities such as vestibular therapy (for dizziness), cognitive rehab apps, and biofeedback devices to track recovery of the autonomic nervous system. Their research-driven approach includes partnerships with the Department of Defense, ensuring stacks are evidence-based and scalable.

Internationally, many other treatment centers integrate advanced tech with holistic care. These treatment centers stack neuromodulation (e.g., electrical stimulation) with physical therapy and psychological support. They share a common thread: they are not afraid to push boundaries, but they do so safely.

Project NEPTUNE 100 was my own way of stacking: extreme isolation with hyperbaric pressure, STEM education, environmental advocacy, and TBI awareness … all in one mission. It showed me that recovery is not linear; it is about layering experiences and therapies to build resilience. If you are reading this and wondering about your next steps, seek out these labs. Start with a consultation at BOL or a similar center so that you can get scanned, formulate a plan, and stack your way to a bolder beginning. Remember, the wreckage is just the start of the rebuild. Your brain has untapped potential; with help, you can unlock it.

CONCLUSION

"Stealing Fire" for TBI Recovery

"The day science begins to study non-physical phenomena, it will make more progress in one decade than in all the previous centuries of its existence."

-Nikola Tesla

BLUF – There is hope for TBI sufferers, but a watershed moment in medicine needs to happen. That is only going to be driven by people changing their paradigm about what we think we can do, and by believing in change. We also discuss my solution for TBI recovery: **Gym, Autophagy, Mindfulness, Telomere lengthening, Hydration, Sleep** (GAMTHS).

Think "BETTER!"
A Brain Injury Recovery Program™

The Think Better Program

The Think Better Program had a total of 13 participants. It sprung from an idea that if people could take one month to care for themselves, they could come out the other side changed for the better. Of the 13 people, I was subject one. After my success, our overall intention was to take a professional or hardcore athlete with TBI and pair him with a former military person who served and had TBI. This created camaraderie and a "buddy" system, where each partner held the other accountable for showing up and being responsible for the actions they took inside the program; they made each other go through it.

You already know that after my radical experiment in treating myself after TBI, I came back stronger than I was before. After completing the Think Better Program, the other 12 members showed improved cognitive function and reduced phase lag. What does that mean? Every single person felt better, thought more quickly, and had a better mood upon completion.

In the Think Better Program, we did everything I discussed in chapter four, and people came to the facility as if it were their job. They spent approximately 8 hours a day for 20 days there (5 days a week, with weekends off). We provided them with support and mentorship and had many discussions.

However, this was not a clinical trial; it was entirely observational. We looked for objective quality measures to verify change, and we observed significant improvements among our participants. Two of the letters that you see in the back of this book are from people who went through the program or their loved ones. The words of affirmation are incredible.

Stealing Fire

"Stealing fire" is a powerful term which refers to the acquisition of knowledge, technology, or insight by defying authority and challenging the status quo. Drawing primarily from the Greek myth of Prometheus, stealing fire has come to represent daring innovation, rebellion, and the pursuit of enlightenment, often at great personal risk.

In mythology, Prometheus, a champion of humanity, defied Zeus, the king of the gods, by stealing fire from Mount Olympus and giving it to the mortals. As punishment for making this gift, which enabled the progress of civilization, Prometheus was sentenced to eternal torment.

Modern-day "Prometheans" are innovators in fields such as technology and science, creating breakthroughs that transform human life. Stealing fire also symbolizes the courage to challenge established norms and conventional wisdom. It is used to describe rebels, activists, or revolutionary thinkers who defy authority to ignite change. On an individual level, "stealing fire" is the pursuit of personal inspiration, self-empowerment, or spiritual awakening. It involves moving past limitations to unlock one's inner passion and transformative knowledge. The concept embodies the human desire to push boundaries and acquire difficult or forbidden knowledge. It acknowledges that such pursuits often come with consequences, much like Prometheus' punishment.

Finding your passion or your personal mission is motivating. At this point, as a TBI survivor, you should be looking for a purpose. Doing so will increase your odds of survival and further your healing journey. Set small goals at first, like going to your child's recital or celebrating a relative's next birthday. Achieving those small goals will grow into a larger purpose, like helping someone get through TBI recovery. Ultimately, you can find purpose in your mission, but knowing your mission will bring you a sense of purpose.

Additionally, finding some sort of community can be cathartic. There are groups of survivors out there; these are people with whom you can share your experience. If you engage and allow yourself to become part of something, you will start to feel better. This group of newfound friends can also help you to try new things. Merely trying to learn something new can be stimulating enough to get your mind flowing. Make your tasks fun and, like my friend always says, "keep it weird." You get one pass at this life, and it is supposed to be enjoyed.

This type of wellness program is "stealing fire." I want to explain how the program works so that everybody will understand its value.

The Results

TBI does not lend itself to discovery by conventional means. As for results, we measured as many objective quality measures as we could. We used 19 psychological and psychosocial tests. The results are summarized in Table 1.[68] The before-and-after scores are profound and show improvement for every participant. Electroencephalographs were performed on all participants before, during, and after the program. The summary Z-score analyses indicates an increase in EEG coherence and a change in sleeping patterns.[69] (See the results in Appendix B).

While the EEG results, coupled with the testing, offer a compelling argument for this therapy, it is no magic pill or

[68] See Table 1 in Appendix B.

[69] See Figures 1, 2, and 3 in Appendix B.

elixir. This program is just a way of feeling better. Every single person has experienced the results they received, although the number was very small. All 13 participants still keep in touch with me regularly. It is such a pleasure to have been able to help people. According to the drug company model, I don't know which treatment was most effective or had the greatest efficacy.

I believe that doing all of the therapies together and taking myself offline for an entire month was key. That sentiment has also been echoed by many of the people in the program. Finally, they had a glimmer of hope and an upward trend, with impressive results. One participant went to a concert, where he saved three people's lives. One participant, a football player, was married to a physician; the wife asked for a sit down with me to hear the mechanisms of action and what I thought was going on scientifically because, she said she had a "changed husband." Most compelling to me are the relationships I made, such as a young lady, the daughter of a participant, who credits me with "saving her dad's life." Another female veteran's daughter still remains in contact with me and sends me presents. I am honored to have their appreciation, and I love my ability to help these people. This is just another reason why I think my TBI was the best thing to ever happen to me.

Importantly, this program need not be a treatment only for TBI; rather, it can be used as a "tune-up" for anyone. I experimented by providing the program for half the time (2 weeks of 8 hours per day, 5 days per week) to a couple of people who were asymptomatic for TBI; after 2 weeks, they had significant improvement in cognitive response as well as an overall feeling of "well-being." I understand these results are not publishable as clinical data, but the individual stories are compelling and provocative. There is hope: we may have control over our future, and we are not doomed. *You must take care of yourself; it is quite literally the most important thing you can do in your life.*

I recognize that hope is not a strategy, but it is a start. I tried to find a way to heal myself and, in doing so, stumbled upon a way to help others. I hope that you can find a program like this, and if not, remember to try different things to help yourself or your loved one feel better without making things worse. Help is within reach. And no, we will not settle for a tincture of time to heal our TBI; we do not need to, because knowledge is power.

Hope for Your TBI

Either you take time now to get your healing going, or you will be forced to make time later. Please, start now. I know so many people, especially people from this program, who struggled with their symptoms daily. Some lived in unnecessary fog. Some experienced extreme anger, yelling at their loved ones. Worse yet, many contemplated suicide, with some even putting a gun in their mouth, and others attempting suicide and thankfully, failing. The program brought them back from the brink. It is crucial to get knowledge in the hands of those suffering so they have hope, and realize change is possible. This is not false hope, but true hope based on real science and mechanisms of action from known primary treatment modalities, as well as adjunctive care modalities. This blend of science, while not completely proven, is a step in the right direction.

All this work to repair TBIs amounts to a great form of a tune-up for all humans. It is what people call biohacking nowadays, but it really is just a new definition of "health care." There is an old saying that seems appropriate in this context: "Those who claim something cannot be done should not interfere with those doing it."

As a researcher and survivor of TBI, I have learned that healing is not a solitary struggle but a collective quest. It is a bold leap into the art of the possible, fueled by passion and a shared mission. You, the reader, are not just holding this book; **you are grasping a torch**, ready to light the way for a revolution in how we understand and treat TBI. The pain of TBI is deeply personal: the residual self-image of who we once were collides with the stark reality of trembling hands, the struggle to read, or legs that refuse to obey. This feels like a betrayal by our own bodies, sparking anger, shame, and a fear of revealing our imperfections, as if a chink in our armor makes us less human. But in this raw vulnerability lies the spark of a movement, a **movement you are now part of, one that redefines healing for every TBI survivor and their loved ones**. And if you are a TBI survivor, send a message loud and clear to any demons, "I FIGHT BACK!" Remember: YOU ARE THE SINGLE MOST INFLUENTIAL PERSON YOU WILL MEET AND TALK TO TODAY AND EVERY DAY!

The modern medical system is a suffocating bureaucracy, chaining doctors to ICD-10 codes and endless paperwork that strip away their ability to truly see their patients. Doctors, ensnared by this broken system, are not just discouraged but actively blocked from forging the human connections that healing requires. They chase a sterile ideal of "perfect," forcing every patient into a one-size-fits-all mold, ignoring the unique needs of each TBI survivor. As I have said before, if you have seen one TBI …you have seen ONE TBI. TBI is not as well understood as you think it is by the "white coats." Perfect is the enemy of "good enough."

If doctors focused on improving lives – physically, physiologically, and psychologically – they would transform medicine. Instead, they are trapped in a machine that values billing over breakthroughs. **Traditional medicine has had thousands of years to solve the TBI puzzle, and despite some progress in the last 50 years, it has failed to deliver a cure.** Drugs, with their grim warnings of nausea, depression, rectal bleeding, or even death, are not the answer; they are merely a shaky stepping stone. The drug company model, which tests one variable at a time, is built on a flawed premise: healing is linear. We must reject this notion and embrace a dynamic, holistic approach that tests and refines combinations of therapies for Constant and Never-Ending Improvement (CANEI).

Advice for TBI Recovery: Gym, Autophagy, Mindfulness, Telomere lengthening, Hydration, Sleep (GAMTHS)

In my own fight with TBI, I have forged an imprecise, battle-tested cocktail of practices that have not only fueled my recovery but reshaped my life and longevity. This is a vague philosophy, with a regimen you can adopt today and then deviate from as you learn and grow on your own journey. I call this regimen **GAMTHS**:

- **Gym Workouts**: Commit to regular exercise to build muscle, enhance balance, strengthen grip, and boost mobility. Each rep is a rebellion against limitation and a ticket to freedom. Grip strength is not just about holding weights, but rather, it is a prime predictor of overall health. Every 11 lbs. (5 kg) decrease in grip strength is linked to a 16% increase in all-cause mortality.[70] Grip strength serves as a vital sign, reflecting muscular endurance, aerobic fitness, flexibility, balance, and coordination, with a weaker grip associated with higher risks of chronic disease and mortality. At the very least, get out and move. They say a body in motion stays in motion.[71]

- **Autophagy (Detox):** Autophagy is your body's self-cleaning mechanism; it breaks down damaged cells or cellular components and recycles components into amino acids and other building blocks for energy and repair, clearing neural debris and reducing inflammation in TBI recovery.[72] Practice intermittent fasting (if supported by your body type and if you don't have a history of eating disorders), eat clean, prioritize high protein, and reduce adipose tissue to cleanse your body at a cellular level.
- **Mindset Mastery**: Cultivate faith, practice meditation, manage cortisol, and pursue relentless personal growth to fortify your spirit against despair. When a loved one whispers "calm down," take the opportunity to breathe. Faith (whether spiritual or rooted in resilience) fosters hope and emotional regulation, reducing anxiety and enhancing well-being. Use apps to make meditation a habit, or just pick a time every day and plan to do it.

[70] Leong. (July 2015).

[71] See Appendix B for more information on exercise, mindfulness, hydration, and sleep.

[72] See Appendix A for more information on clean eating and intermittent fasting.

A common complaint is, "I'm too busy to meditate." I opine that the busiest people are the ones in need of meditation the most. As Mahatma Gandhi famously said, "I have so much to accomplish today that I must meditate for two hours instead of one." Keep in mind that you are the most important and influential person with whom you will speak today and every day!

- **Telomere Lengthening**: Use HBOT and eliminate processed and ultra-processed foods to support DNA transcription and cellular vitality.
- **Hydration**: Chronic dehydration, often mistaken for fatigue in the 3 p.m. lull of the day, plagues most people. Drink water relentlessly to fuel cellular health. Hydration maintains electrolyte balance (sodium, potassium, magnesium), which regulates nerve function, muscle contractions, and pH balance, preventing cramps, fatigue, and cognitive issues during TBI recovery. Hydrate with about a gallon (3 to 4 liters) of water daily, adjusting intake for activity.
- **Sleep**: Sleep is the cornerstone of healing; if you cannot sleep, you cannot heal. Work at good sleep hygiene like it is your job. Quality sleep (7 to 9 hours) facilitates tissue repair, hormone release (e.g., growth hormone for regeneration), immune function, reduces inflammation, and supports TBI recovery. Practice consistent schedules, dark rooms, no screens before bed, and relaxation techniques. That phone is not your friend, and I could write a whole book on people not being able to put it down; please, one hour before bed, plug it in in another room and pretend it is not there.

Advice for Recovery

1. **Exercise:** As previously mentioned, working out can also induce hormesis. Gym routines should also target stabilizer muscles, critical for preventing falls, a leading cause of injury and death in older adults. Balance and strength training reduces the risk of falls in older people.[73] Workouts increase blood flow, elevating vascular endothelial growth factor (VEGF) levels, which drive angiogenesis (the formation of new blood vessels) to improve tissue repair and oxygen delivery, which are both essential for TBI recovery. Exercise also boosts interleukin-15 (IL-15), a myokine with antimicrobial and anti-inflammatory properties that supports immune function, reduces inflammation, and enhances skin healing and anti-tumor immunity, acting as a natural "antibiotic." Incorporate compound movements like deadlifts and rows 3 to 5 times per week.
2. **Autophagy Activation**: The mechanistic target of rapamycin (mTOR) is a protein kinase that acts like a switch controlling cellular processes, including autophagy. Autophagy is inhibited by mTOR. It also suppresses autophagy-related protein expression, prioritizing growth over cellular recycling. When fasting or in a caloric deficit, mTOR activity decreases, allowing autophagy to restore cellular homeostasis. You need a balance between the two processes. If your body is constantly feeding, you are not doing the cleanup portion, and if you are constantly doing the cleanup portion, you are not building.

---

[73] Sherrington. (November 2016),.

3. **Clean eating and intermittent fasting**: Start with supervised intermittent fasting if your body type supports it and build gradually if needed. Intermittent fasting (e.g., the 16:8 method, in which you consume food only during an 8 hour window per day, and fast for the remaining 16 hours) triggers autophagy, promoting longevity, anti-aging, and protection against neurodegeneration. Focus on clean eating (whole foods like vegetables, lean meats, and nuts). Increased protein intake supports muscle preservation and autophagic flux. Excess body fat hinders autophagy and contributes to metabolic disorders. Decreasing adipose tissue (fat) reduces toxins stored in fat cells, thereby amplifying detoxification and weight loss. This practice regenerates healthier cells and boosts energy for sustained TBI healing, outperforming fad diets.
4. **Mindset Mastery:** Meditation, even 10–15 minutes daily, lowers cortisol by up to 25%, improving focus, self-awareness, and emotional health while slowing mental aging and supporting immunity. Stress management through deep breathing prevents chronic cortisol elevation, which worsens TBI symptoms like inflammation and cognitive fog. Personal growth via journaling or goal-setting builds a growth mindset, enhancing flexibility, concentration, and self-compassion, turning setbacks into opportunities. These elements reduce depression risk and promote telomere preservation and immune health.
5. **Lengthen Telomeres:** Telomeres (protective caps on chromosomes) shorten with age and stress, accelerating

TBI-related decline; HBOT increases telomere length by over 20% in immune cells through repeated sessions, clearing aged cells. Protocols with 60 daily sessions (over the course of many months) at 2.0 atmospheres improve cognition, performance, and anti-aging markers. Avoiding processed foods (>3 servings/day) is critical, as they're linked to shorter telomeres, faster aging, and higher risks of obesity, cancer, and diabetes. Diets high in saturated fats, sugars, and additives exacerbate telomere attrition, while whole foods preserve telomere length and support DNA repair. Combine HBOT with a clean diet for TBI resilience.

6. **Hydration**: Electrolytes enhance rehydration, support heart health, and boost performance by retaining water and replenishing sweat losses. Use natural sources like coconut water for these "correct chemicals." Removing neurotoxins like fluoride, linked to lower IQ and cognitive deficits at low levels (<1.5 mg/L), is vital, as excess exposure causes neurotoxicity and developmental issues. Use reverse osmosis or distillation to eliminate fluoride, reducing risks of arthritis, bone fractures, and neuropsychiatric effects.
7. **Sleep:** Deep sleep stages consolidate memories, process emotions, and clear toxins via the glymphatic system, preventing cognitive decline. Sleep lowers cortisol, aids weight management, and bolsters immunity, with poor sleep linked to heart disease, diabetes, and delayed wound healing. For TBI, sleep enhances neuroplasticity and recovery from severe injuries.

These practices are not a dismissal of approved therapies but a powerful alternative when the system fails you. You have the absolute right, authority, and responsibility to seize control of your healing when conventional methods fall short.

This journey demands radical acceptance. This trait is not just desired but vital for sanity and recovery. When life gives you lemons, do NOT… make lemonade; learn to love lemons. TBI changes you irrevocably, and resisting that truth only deepens the pain. As Ernest Hemingway said, "There is nothing noble in being superior to your fellow man; true nobility is being superior to your former self."

In my darkest hours after my TBI, I stood at the edge of despair, feeling as if part of me had to die. The weight of that impending loss was crushing, and I contemplated a permanent end, believing no other path existed. As Aeschylus wrote, "In our sleep, pain which cannot forget falls drop by drop upon the heart until, in our own despair, against our will, comes wisdom through the awful grace of God." That wisdom, born of suffering, taught me that it was not my entire self that needed to die; just the parts that no longer served me. The finality of such a choice is irreversible, but there is always another way. Radical acceptance allowed me to release who I was and build who I could become, and it can do the same for you.

You are now part of a movement, a revolution to redefine TBI care and wellness itself. This is bigger than any one of us, and your role is critical. We need new measures of effectiveness that include families, and we need to track changes from pre-injury baselines to a new normal. Research must abandon the outdated drug company model for a holistic approach that treats the entire person, mind, body, and spirit, simultaneously.

This revolution starts with you. Put your pack down for a moment. When was the last time you paused to heal yourself? A brief rest, time to rejuvenate, empowers you to carry more, do more, be more. Join us in this fight. Share your story, advocate for change, and demand better from a system that has let TBI survivors down for too long.

Together, we can win the hearts and minds of others, shift the paradigm, and forge a future where healing is not about reclaiming the past but embracing a better version of ourselves. Our lives are marked by the choices we make. We hear echoes of steps not made, a passage not taken, a door not opened. T.S. Elliot reference aside, I implore you: open that door. Who knows, it may lead to a rose garden.

Here is what I know: life will test you. It will push you to your limits... Some days you'll feel like you've got nothing left... like the weight of the world is pressing down on your chest, and no matter how hard you fight, it's never enough. I FELT THAT TOO.

Listen to me.... You are stronger than this moment! Think hard about every challenge you've already faced. You made it through. Even on the nights I cried myself to sleep, I still woke up and kept moving. You can, too... You did not come this far just to quit now!

This is where most people stop, but you are not most people! You don't give up: you rise, and you push forward. One day you'll look back at this moment and see... not the pain... but the pride it took to move forward. So, take a breath, wipe your tears, and keep going! Your story isn't over; it's just getting started!

Call to Action: Stand with us. Commit to this or some other regimen of healing practices. Spread the word to other survivors, families, and communities. Challenge doctors to see you or your TBI survivor as a person, not an ICD-10 code. Advocate for research that treats the whole person. Start today… Take one step, whether it's a gym session, a glass of water, or a moment of meditation. Share this movement on social media platforms, connect with others, and demand a new normal for TBI care. You are not just a survivor; you are a revolutionary. Together, we will change medicine, rewrite the story of TBI, and prove that resilience is our greatest weapon. Join the movement. The time is now.

ACKNOWLEDGMENTS

I want to acknowledge every person who has ever entered my life. Those who lifted me up and those who knocked me down. BOTH were necessary. The kindness I received gave me strength, and the pain I endured gave me wisdom. Without the full spectrum of these experiences, I would not be the man I am today, nor would I have been able to write this book.

To my family, friends, and the many professionals who supported me through my recovery, THANK YOU! To those whose actions caused me pain or forced me to confront difficult truths, I would like to thank you as well. You were part of the curriculum I needed.

I would also like to specifically thank Linda Bond, a fellow author, for without her this project never would have started.

Most of all, I acknowledge the traumatic brain injury that changed everything. What once felt like the end of my life became the beginning of a deeper, more meaningful one. I am grateful for the breaking, and I am grateful for the rebuilding.

APPENDIX A

TBI Recovery: Gut Health, Diet, Hydration, Sleep, and Mindfulness

1. Severe dysbiosis: This condition is linked to worse neurological outcomes. TBI disrupts vagal signaling and ENS function, causing constipation or diarrhea. Constipation increases toxin reabsorption, worsening neuroinflammation.
2. Ketogenic diet (KD): Emerging research underscores KD's potential in improving cognitive functions and regulating mood. By altering the gut microbiota and its metabolites, the KD may have a positive role in maintaining normal cognitive function and regulating mood, especially in the treatment of neurological disorders and depression. Another study showed that a Ketogenic diet alleviated anxiety and depression associated with insulin-dependent diabetes management.
3. Fermented food: A diet rich in fiber, prebiotics, and fermented foods can promote a healthy, diverse microbiota, while diets high in fat, sugar, and processed foods may contribute to an imbalance that negatively impacts gut and systemic health. Given the gut

microbiota's significant role in the brain–gut axis and immune function, dietary choices are vital for optimizing both physical and mental well-being.

4. Hydration and gut massage: Water prevents constipation, which is common post-TBI. Additionally, try to get your water filtered because of all the chemicals in today's water supply. Importantly, consuming water consistently and adding gut massage, enhances peristalsis (wave-like muscle contractions that move food through the digestive tract).
5. Abdominal massage: This treatment ameliorates insomnia and increases sleep duration. The effect is associated with the regulation of brain-gut peptide levels and the restoration of gut microbiota diversity and structure. These findings suggest that the microbiota-gut-brain axis may be involved in the therapeutic mechanism of abdominal massage for insomnia.
6. On sleep: The glymphatic system (a system of structures and processes that allows soluble waste substances to pass from the cerebrospinal fluid into the surrounding tissue fluid for removal) is constantly filtering toxins from the brain, but during the waking hours, this system remains mainly disengaged. Sleep is one way to engage the glymphatic system and drain toxins from the brain. When the body gets deep sleep, and during REM sleep, the glymphatic system drains almost twice as many proteins as when awake. It is imperative to get deep and REM sleep.
7. Intermittent fasting (additional information and warnings): For TBI patients, intermittent fasting reduces

neuroinflammation and enhances gut-brain axis function by fostering microbial diversity and stimulating ketone production, which aids neuronal repair. While there is a great deal of information online about this, beware: serious fasting requires medical oversight to prevent nutrient deficiencies or exacerbation of HPA axis dysregulation, given TBI-related metabolic vulnerabilities. From fasting, I have personally experienced great clarity after brain fog, and fasting has helped alleviate some of my gut issues. Approaches include time-restricted eating (e.g., eating only within a daily 8-hour window), alternate-day fasting, the 5:2 method (normal eating for five days, then 500–600 calories for two days), and periodic or whole-day fasting.

8. Mindfulness and The Central Nervous System (CNS): The CNS, comprising the brain and spinal cord, orchestrates cognitive and emotional responses. Chronic stress activates the hypothalamic-pituitary-adrenal (HPA) axis, leading to elevated cortisol levels, which can impair neural repair, disrupt immune function, and exacerbate inflammation. Meditation, particularly mindfulness-based techniques, has been shown to downregulate HPA axis activity, thereby reducing cortisol secretion and mitigating these adverse effects. For instance, a 2013 meta-analysis found that mindfulness meditation programs significantly reduced cortisol levels in stressed populations, with effect sizes comparable to pharmacological interventions. The ANS, which regulates involuntary bodily functions such as heart rate, respiration, and digestion, is divided into

the sympathetic nervous system (SNS) and parasympathetic nervous system (PNS). Chronic stress often results in SNS dominance, triggering the "fight-or-flight" response, which elevates heart rate and diverts resources from non-essential functions like digestion. Meditation activates the PNS, promoting a "rest-and-digest" state that counteracts SNS hyperactivity. Studies using heart rate variability (HRV) as a biomarker of ANS balance demonstrate that mindfulness practices increase parasympathetic tone, enhancing cardiovascular health and emotional regulation. For example, a 2018 study showed that a 10-day mindfulness retreat significantly increased HRV, indicating improved PNS activity.

9. Mindfulness and meditation: I approach mindfulness and meditation not only as practices for mental well-being but also as powerful tools for modulating the interplay between the Central Nervous System (CNS), the Autonomic Nervous System (ANS), and the enteric nervous system (ENS). Meditation, a cornerstone of mindfulness, is a scientifically supported method for reducing stress and fostering resilience by influencing these neural networks.
10. Mindfulness studies: Peer-reviewed studies, such as those by Kabat-Zinn on MBSR, provide robust evidence for the efficacy of practicing mindfulness. While I am not a clinical expert in mindfulness, my professional and personal experiences compel me to advocate for its study and application, given its measurable impact on reducing stress, improving neural function,

and aiding in neural repair. It also enhances overall physiological resilience, making it a critical tool for managing the demands of modern life.

11. Reduce toxins: TBI may increase systemic toxin load, as neuroinflammation and gut permeability allow harmful substances to accumulate. Toxins can accumulate in various parts of the body, with some of the most common storage locations being the liver, kidneys, fatty tissues, and blood. Dietary toxins like processed foods, environmental exposures such as pesticides, and stress pollute the body, disrupting the gut microbiome and worsening TBI outcomes. As previously stated, skip central-aisle products with emulsifiers or sugars that promote dysbiosis (the imbalance in the different microorganisms living together in the gut). Choose organic produce and filtered water to limit pesticides and heavy metals, which impair gut barriers. Meditation and yoga lower cortisol, supporting gut health. These steps create a clean environment for gut healing, critical for TBI patients.
12. HBOT: Hyperbaric oxygen therapy (HBOT) inhibits toxin activity and enhances oxygenation, supporting neural repair. Binding agents, such as bentonite clay or activated charcoal, absorb toxins in the GI tract, reducing systemic burden. These interventions require medical supervision to avoid nutrient depletion or interactions with medications.
13. Reduce plastic byproduct consumption: Plastics are widely used for food and water storage. These can release harmful toxins like bisphenol A (BPA), phthalates, and

microplastics, which leach into contents, especially under heat or over time. Your plastic water bottle sat in a truck and heated up on its way to your hands, regardless of how cold it is now. In contrast, materials like glass, stainless steel, or ceramic are inert, minimizing chemical leaching and ensuring safer storage. Choosing these alternatives for drinking, eating, cooking, and storing food reduces exposure to toxic substances, promoting better health outcomes based on current scientific evidence.

APPENDIX B

Results for The Think Better Program

1. Normally, I would have looked at an MRI with Diffusion Tensor Imaging (DTI). However, no studies have shown an increase in blood flow associated with a cured TBI. So, we used measures such as 19 psychological and psychosocial tests. The composite scores from psychological and psychosocial testing are summarized in Table 1 (below).

Patient Profile	Percentile Range				> 74	25 - 74	9 - 24	2 - 8	< 2
	Standard Score Range				> 109	90 - 109	80 - 89	70 - 79	< 70
Domain Scores	Patient Score	Standard Score	Percentile	VI**	Above	Average	Low Average	Low	Very Low
Composite Memory	89	83	13	Yes			X		
Verbal Memory	43	71	3	Yes				X	
Visual Memory	46	103	58	Yes		X			
Reaction Time*	703	95	37	Yes		X			

Psychological Profile testing BEFORE treatment

Patient Profile	Percentile Range				> 74	25 - 74	9 - 24	2 - 8	< 2
	Standard Score Range				> 109	90 - 109	80 - 89	70 - 79	< 7
Domain Scores	Patient Score	Standard Score	Percentile	VI**	Above	Average	Low Average	Low	Ver Low
Composite Memory	99	104	61	Yes		X			
Verbal Memory	54	106	66	Yes		X			
Visual Memory	45	100	50	Yes		X			
Executive Function	67	131	98	Yes	X				

Psychological Profile testing AFTER treatment

2. Additionally, electroencephalographs were performed on all participants before, during, and after.

The summary Z-score analysis, as shown in Figure 1 (below), indicates an increase in EEG coherence, which is often used to assess functional connectivity in the human cortex. Moreover, a sharp decrease in phase lag is also noted. This is profound because it shows the brain is increasing its speed and connectivity. Figures 2 and 3 represent theta and gamma z-score reductions, indicating a change in sleeping patterns (in the case of Theta) as well as a change in multiprocessing capacity (in the case of Gamma).

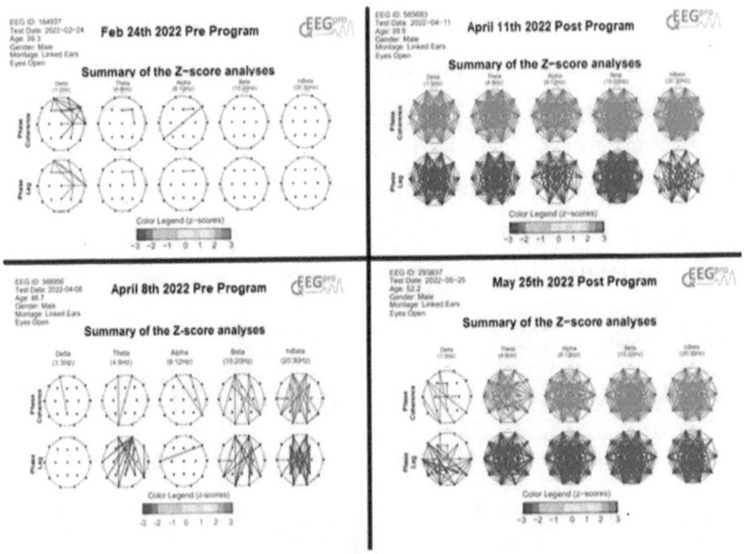

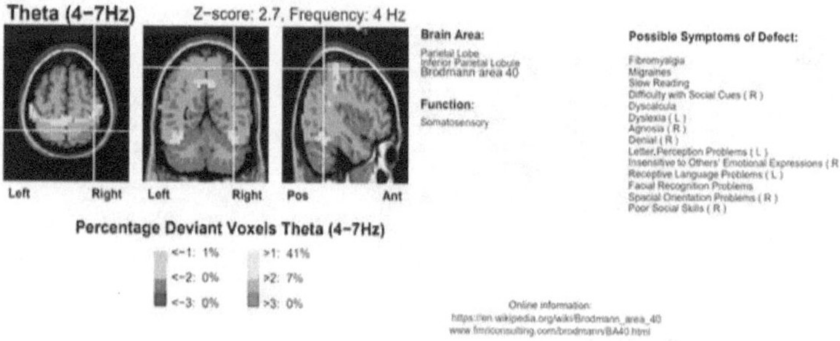

BEFORE Treatment

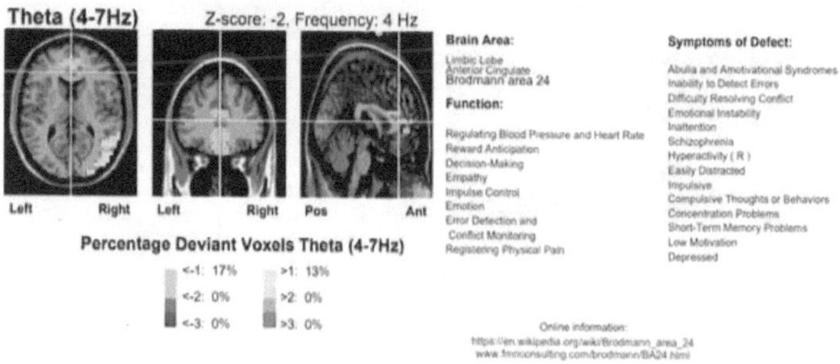

AFTER Treatment

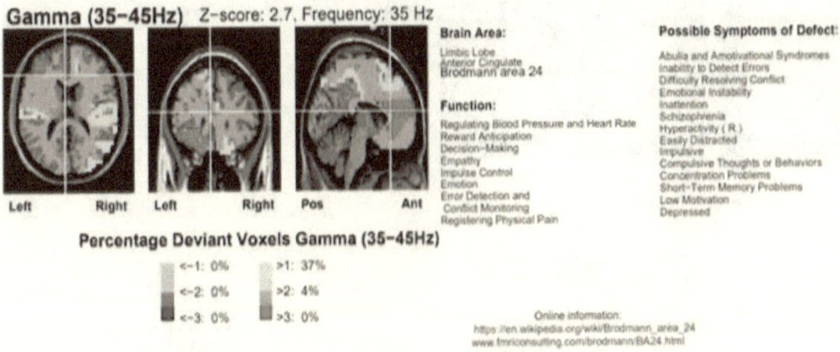

BEFORE Treatment

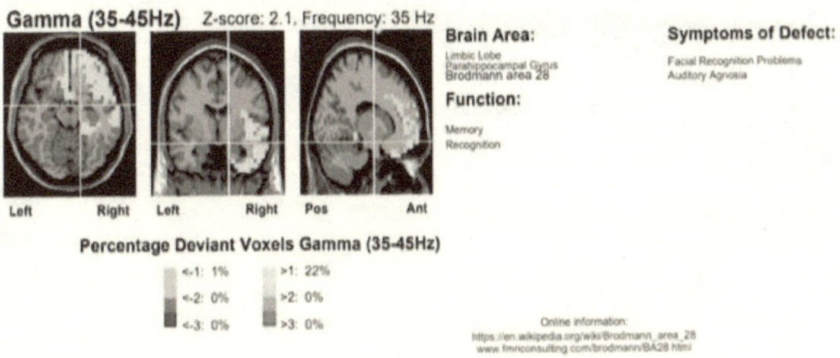

AFTER Treatment

APPENDIX C

Letters in Support of a New Way to Heal

From: Nicole ddddddd < ddddddd@hotmail.com>
Sent: Wednesday, May 22, 2024 11:26:14 AM
To: Dr. Joseph Dituri, CDR, USN (ret) <joe@gallantaquatic.com>
Subject: Michael ddddddd - progress
Good morning,

I hope this e-mail finds both of you well. I 've been holding my breath for two months now (since Mike left the Tampa clinic) thinking that he would start to revert back to his erratic behaviors before he left. Believe me when I say that YOU have both saved our lives and feel like I'm getting back the man that I married 18 years ago.

Before the clinic, Mike had some good days, but the bad days certainly outweighed them. I felt like I was raising a third child. He would become argumentative, volatile, and would perseverate over so many things. At one point, I finally understood what it must feel like to be exposed to extreme emotional abuse. If he couldn't handle something, I would find him upstairs hiding under his pillow, and sometimes this would last for days on end. He was unable to sleep. At times, he didn't understand the point of going to work anymore. He hated strangers, he hated friends, he hated family. In January, I was at my breaking point and considering divorce. Not because I don't love him more than anyone, but because I simply couldn't take the emotional abuse and extreme behaviors that were happening around our kids. I knew it was his TBI symptoms, but the days were becoming intolerable.

I've read so many books in the last 18 months about brain injury so that I could better understand. I made sure he had cognitive therapy, regular exercise, plenty of rest, access to a neuropsychiatrist, visits with a nutritionist when he couldn't remember to eat. He went to 3 different therapists and checked himself out every time (when the topics became too deep/personal). Almost 2 ½ years went by and I felt like we were spinning our wheels.

When I finally found a way to pay for your program, I called in February and I'm forever grateful that I did. He now reports that he feels like a different person, almost better than before. His anxiety is now minimal, his energy is up, and his reasoning is so much better. I feel like I am speaking to a reasonable and understanding adult again. Thank you, thank you, thank you.

Dr. (therapist), I hope you will continue to work with Mike and peel back some of those layers that challenge him. When life stresses him out, I still notice that he tends to drink more than he should, but he is consciously working on it (choosing low ABV beer). I hope you can continue to talk to him about this regularly and help him find better ways to cope with difficult situations.

Again, I thank you for the work you do, and I, along with all of our family, thanks you.

Kind regards,
Nicole dddddd

Dr. Dituri, his program, and his team literally saved my life. I don't say that lightly or as a cliche either.

I had played a college sport that had a high concussion rate to it. Unbeknownst to me, I'd sustained a lot of concussions. A lot of times, people will think those are the major ones where your arm goes straight, but it appears that in recent studies, the little ones—the ones where you see stars—do quite a bit of harm also.

I'd gotten to a point in life where things started going downhill dramatically. Some people would say that it's old age, but I knew something was different. I'd tried many things, but to no avail.

When I contacted Dr. Dituri, he was completely confident in his program and the effects that it could have on a traumatic brain injury. After going through his program, I understand why he was so confident.

Now, I'll be honest—it wasn't easy. But I guess you could say all the years of concussions and brain injury weren't easy either. The program was life-changing. The combination of hyperbaric oxygen chamber therapy, neurofeedback, and a whole assortment of supportive treatments—the program was literally able to work miracles.

I remember the first time that I noticed this miracle, and it was relatively early on in the process. After about three or four days of being in the program, I wound up hitting a massive amount of traffic on the way in that morning. It was so massive that many roads were closed off and people were trying to find other routes, which caused what turned out to be about an hour-and-twenty-minute delay on a forty-minute trip.

I used the GPS, rerouted multiple times, and eventually made it to the program headquarters. I pulled over to the side of the road to decompress for what I thought would be fifteen minutes—where I would have fifteen minutes of yelling and screaming in frustration, trying to calm myself down and gather my thoughts.

But as I pulled over, I realized I wasn't stressed. I hadn't wasted a full day's worth of energy on one ride. My massive anxiety and frustration had subsided. I was calm. I was resolute. I was ready to go in and start the training.

This was completely and absolutely new territory for me. Normally, I would've been shot for the whole day—all energy would've been drained from my body, and I would've made new enemies with my bad temper. But not today. Today, life was different. I was calm, I handled the situation with logic, and I was ready to proceed with the rest of the training.

-Greg W.

DETAILED GLOSSARY OF TERMS FROM "SHATTERED TO STRONG"

This glossary provides thorough definitions for all difficult, technical, or commonly misunderstood terms appearing in "Shattered to Strong." Terms are drawn from the entire document. Definitions are based on standard scientific, medical, and contextual meanings, with explanations tailored to their usage in the proposal for clarity. Terms are listed alphabetically for ease of reference.

Aeschylus. An ancient Greek tragedian (c. 525-456 BCE) known for plays like *Agamemnon*. In the proposal, referenced for a quote on wisdom through suffering: "In our sleep, pain which cannot forget falls drop by drop upon the heart until, in our own despair, against our will, comes wisdom through the awful grace of God." A major theme of this book is that you can grow from adversity.

Allopathic Medicine. The conventional Western medical approach focused on treating symptoms and diseases using drugs, surgery, and other interventions that counteract the effects of illness. Contrasted in the proposal with holistic or alternative methods, criticized as having "lost its way" and being influenced by the pharmaceutical industry.

Angiogenesis. The physiological process of forming new blood vessels from pre-existing ones. In TBI recovery, it improves tissue repair and oxygen delivery, stimulated by practices like gym workouts, HBOT, and WBV therapy via elevated VEGF levels.

Antagonist Muscle Groups. Muscles that oppose the action of agonist muscles (e.g., biceps vs. triceps). Imbalances between them can lead to mobility issues in TBI; reciprocal inhibition helps restore balance through targeted exercises.

Assiduousness. Diligent and persistent effort or attention to detail. Listed in the proposal as a personal value for TBI recovery, emphasizing consistent application of healing practices.

Astronautical Engineering. The branch of engineering focused on the design, development, and operation of spacecraft and related systems. The author's master's degree topic, with a thesis on orbital determination and life support systems.

Atmospheric Diving System. A one-person submersible suit allowing deep-sea diving without decompression, certified to 2000 feet of seawater. The author oversaw its certification during Navy service.

Autophagy. The body's cellular self-cleaning mechanism that breaks down and recycles damaged components for energy and repair. Crucial for TBI by clearing neural debris and reducing inflammation; activated through detox, fasting, clean eating, high protein, and reducing adipose tissue.

BDNF (Brain-Derived Neurotrophic Factor). A protein promoting neuron survival, growth, and synapse formation. Enhanced by cold exposure (e.g., ice baths), exercise, and nature exposure; supports neuroplasticity and TBI recovery by increasing hippocampal neurogenesis.

Bemer™ Mat. A device for pulsed electromagnetic field (PEMF) therapy, delivering electromagnetic pulses to stimulate cellular repair and reduce inflammation. Used off-label for TBI to improve mitochondrial function and neurogenesis.

BFR (Blood Flow Restriction) Therapy. See KAATSU Band Therapy.

Biohacking. The practice of using science, technology, and lifestyle changes to optimize human biology and performance. In the proposal, reframed as a "new definition of healthcare" through modalities like HBOT, ice baths, and neurofeedback for TBI recovery.

Biomedical Engineering. An interdisciplinary field applying engineering principles to medicine and biology for healthcare innovations. The author's PhD focus, with research in life support equipment, high CO2 environments, hyperbaric, and hypobaric medicine.

BLUF (Bottom Line Up Front). A military briefing technique providing the key conclusion or overview at the start of a discussion. Used in the proposal to structure chapters for clarity on complex TBI topics.

Blue Blockers. Eyewear or filters that block blue light from screens to improve sleep hygiene by reducing melatonin suppression. Recommended in the proposal for better rest during TBI recovery.

Brain Optimization Lab (BOL). A cutting edge treatment facility that specializes in addressing catastrophic injuries like TBI and CTE through a multidisciplinary approach.

CANEI (Constant and Never-Ending Improvement). A mindset of perpetual self-betterment, applied to TBI by continuously challenging oneself and modulating therapies. Emphasizes avoiding complacency for ongoing progress.

Center of Excellence for Aging and Brain Repair. A research center at USF's Morsani Medical College focusing on neurodegenerative diseases and brain injury. The author's affiliation for TBI research in veterans' health.

Cerebrolysin. A neuropeptide preparation used off-label for neuroprotection in TBI. Promotes cognitive recovery by supporting neuroplasticity and reducing oxidative stress.

Chiropractic Care. Manual adjustment of the spine to improve nervous system function, alignment, and mobility. For TBI, it reduces neuroinflammation, improves cerebrospinal fluid flow, and complements breathing techniques.

Cold-Shock Protein. Proteins like RBM3 induced by hypothermia (e.g., ice baths), protecting neurons and promoting neurogenesis in brain injuries. References highlight its role in modulating YAP mRNA stability and reducing inflammation.

Cortisol. A glucocorticoid hormone released in response to stress, regulating metabolism and immune response. Chronic elevation worsens TBI symptoms; managed through meditation, faith, and personal growth in mindset mastery.

Deep Submergence Unit (DSU). A U.S. Navy unit specializing in deep-sea rescue and recovery operations. The author served as Officer-in-Charge, earning awards for excellence.

Edwin Smith Papyrus. An ancient Egyptian medical text (c. 1600 BCE) describing head injuries and symptoms, representing early recognition of TBI in historical literature.

Electrolyte Balance. The maintenance of minerals like sodium, potassium, and magnesium in body fluids for nerve function, muscle contractions, and pH regulation. Essential in hydration for TBI to prevent fatigue and cognitive impairment.

GAMTHS. My advice for TBI Recovery: Gym, Autophagy, Mindfulness, Telomere lengthening, Hydration, Sleep.

Glymphatic System. The brain's waste clearance pathway, active during sleep, that removes toxins via cerebrospinal fluid flow. Critical for preventing cognitive decline in TBI; enhanced by quality sleep.

Grounding (Earthing). Direct physical contact with the Earth to absorb electrons, reducing inflammation and oxidative stress. Combined with facing east for sunrise to regulate circadian rhythms in TBI recovery.

HBOT (Hyperbaric Oxygen Therapy). Breathing pure oxygen in a pressurized chamber to increase tissue oxygenation. Supports telomere lengthening, mitochondrial biogenesis, reduces inflammation, and promotes TBI repair; used in the author's recovery.

Hypobaric Medicine. The study of medical effects from low atmospheric pressure environments (e.g., high altitudes or space). Part of the author's PhD research.

Hyperbaric Medicine. The medical use of high atmospheric pressure, often with oxygen, to treat conditions like decompression sickness and TBI. The author's expertise, including co-authoring a book on the topic.

ICD-10 Codes. The 10th revision of the International Classification of Diseases, used for diagnosing and billing. Criticized in the proposal for hindering personalized TBI care due to bureaucratic focus.

IL-15 (Interleukin-15). A cytokine boosted by exercise, with anti-inflammatory and antimicrobial effects. Acts as a natural antibiotic, supporting immune function in TBI recovery.

International Board of Undersea Medicine. An organization certifying undersea medical practices. The author serves as chairman.

John Hughlings Jackson. A 19th-century neurologist who studied brain trauma's neurological impacts, contributing to early modern understanding of TBI.

Jules Undersea Lab. An underwater habitat in Key Largo, Florida, where the author lived for 100 days to study pressurization effects and promote STEM/ocean conservation.

KAATSU Band Therapy. Blood flow restriction training using cuffs to enhance muscle growth and hormone release with low-intensity exercise. Boosts VEGF and nitric oxide for cerebral blood flow in TBI.

Mitochondrial Biogenesis. The process of increasing mitochondrial number and function in cells. Promoted by HBOT and exercise, improving energy production and resilience in TBI-affected brains.

Morsani Medical College. The medical school at the University of South Florida, where the author is an assistant professor of practice.

mTOR (mechanistic Target of Rapamycin). A signaling pathway regulating cell growth and metabolism. Inhibited by autophagy for cleanup; balanced in longevity and TBI for repair vs. building; constant feeding activates it, hindering cleanup.

Neurofeedback. Biofeedback training using EEG to self-regulate brain activity. Improves cognitive and emotional function in TBI by enhancing neuroplasticity.

Neuromuscular Imbalance. Disrupted coordination between muscles and nerves, often in TBI due to injury. Leads to agonist-antagonist imbalances; addressed through exercise and reciprocal inhibition.

Neuroplasticity. The brain's capacity to reorganize neural pathways in response to injury or experience. Key to TBI recovery, supported by sleep, BDNF, and therapies like HBOT and neurofeedback.

Occipital Lobe Massage. Manual stimulation of the brain's visual processing area to potentially reduce tension and support recovery. Used in the author's TBI plan as an alternative therapy.

PEMF (Pulsed Electromagnetic Field) Therapy. See Bemer™ Mat.

Project NEPTUNE 100. The author's 100-day underwater mission to study isolation, pressurization, STEM education, and ocean conservation while advancing TBI research.

PTSD (Post-Traumatic Stress Disorder). A psychiatric disorder from trauma, with symptoms like anxiety and flashbacks. Often co-occurs with TBI; the author's research focus for veterans.

Quo Vadis. Latin for "Where are you going?" Used in the proposal to emphasize keeping the end goal in mind, popularized by Deming in quality management.

Radical Acceptance. Fully embracing reality without resistance, required for TBI sanity and recovery. Involves accepting irrevocable changes to foster growth.

RBM3 (RNA-Binding Motif Protein 3). A protective protein induced by cold stress, associated with neurogenesis and reduced inflammation in TBI. References show its role in modulating mRNA stability and stroke outcomes.

Reciprocal Inhibition. Used in therapy to correct neuromuscular imbalances in TBI for better mobility.

Shake Plate. See WBV (Whole Body Vibration) Therapy.

STEM Education. Science, Technology, Engineering, and Mathematics education. Promoted in Project NEPTUNE 100 to inspire youth.

Submarine Rescue Diving & Recompression System. A Navy system for underwater rescue, designed by the author for transfer under pressure saturation diving.

Superman Pose. A power pose (standing tall with hands on hips) to raise testosterone and confidence. Referenced from Harvard studies on postural effects on hormones.

TBI (Traumatic Brain Injury). Brain dysfunction from external force, ranging from mild concussions to severe damage. Central to the book, with the author's personal experience driving alternative recovery methods.

Telomere Lengthening. Extending chromosome end-caps to delay cellular aging. Achieved via HBOT and avoiding processed foods; supports DNA repair and vitality in TBI.

VEGF (Vascular Endothelial Growth Factor). A protein signaling angiogenesis. Elevated by exercise, HBOT, and KAATSU for improved blood vessel formation and brain repair in TBI.

WBV (Whole Body Vibration) Therapy. Vibration platform exercises (20–50 Hz) to stimulate muscles and neurons. Reduces neuroinflammation and enhances motor function in TBI, accessible for mobility-limited individuals.

William Edwards Deming. An American engineer (1900–1993) known as the father of quality management. Popularized "keep the end in mind" and influenced the BLUF technique.

BIBLIOGRAPHY

Amjad, Imran, Imran Khan Niazi, Nitika Kumari, Usman Ghani, Usman Rashid, Felipe Coutinho Duarte, Federico Fortuna, et al. "The Effects of 12 Weeks of Chiropractic Spinal Adjustments on Physiological Biomarkers in Adults: A Pragmatic Randomized Controlled Trial." PLOS One 20, no. 12 (December 11, 2025). https://doi.org/10.1371/journal.pone.0338730.

Anderson, Kelly E., Nathorn Chaiyakunapruk, Eric J. Gutierrez, H. Weston Schmutz, Michael R. Rose, Diana Brixner, and R. Brett McQueen. "State Out-of-Pocket Caps on Insulin Costs: No Significant Increase in Claims or Utilization." Health Affairs 43, no. 8 (August 1, 2024): 1137–46. https://doi.org/10.1377/hlthaff.2024.00118.

Bakshi, Arjun. "Biochemistry, Serotonin." StatPearls [Internet]., October 5, 2022. https://www.ncbi.nlm.nih.gov/books/NBK560856/

Baquedano, Constanza, Antonia Olguí, Luis Sebastian Contreras-Huerta, Fernando E. Rosas, and Mar Estarellas. "Your Brain on Nature: A Scoping Review of the Neuroscience of Nature Exposure." Neuroscience & Biobehavioral Reviews 183 (April 2026): 106565. https://doi.org/10.1016/j.neubiorev.2026.106565.

Berding, Kirsten, Klara Vlckova, Wolfgang Marx, Harriet Schellekens, Catherine Stanton, Gerard Clarke, Felice Jacka, Timothy G Dinan, and John F Cryan. "Diet and the Microbiota–Gut–Brain Axis: Sowing the Seeds of Good Mental Health." Advances in Nutrition 12, no. 4 (March 9, 2021): 1239–85. https://doi.org/10.1093/advances/nmaa181.

Bergold PJ, Furhang R, Lawless S. Treating Traumatic Brain Injury with Minocycline. Neurotherapeutics. 2023 Oct;20(6):1546-1564. doi: 10.1007/s13311-023-01426-9. Epub 2023 Sep 18. PMID: 37721647; PMCID: PMC10684850.

"Researchers Find CTE in 345 of 376 Former NFL Players Studied." Boston University Chobanian & Avedisian School of Medicine, 2023. https://www.bumc.bu.edu/camed/2023/02/06/researchers-find-cte-in-345-of-376-former-nfl-players-studied.

Breault, Joseph L, and Emily Knafl. "Pitfalls and Safeguards in Industry-Funded Research." Ochsner Journal, 2020. https://pmc.ncbi.nlm.nih.gov/articles/PMC7122252/.

Cao, Shuqiang, Manrui Li, Yuwen Sun, Peiyan Wu, Wenjie Yang, Hao Dai, Yadong Guo, et al. "Intermittent Fasting Enhances Hippocampal NPY Expression to Promote Neurogenesis after Traumatic Brain Injury." Nutrition 97 (May 2022): 111621. https://doi.org/10.1016/j.nut.2022.111621.

Carter KS, Carter R 3rd. Breath-based meditation: A mechanism to restore the physiological and cognitive reserves for optimal human performance. World J Clin Cases. 2016 Apr 16;4(4):99-102. doi: 10.12998/wjcc.v4.i4.99. PMID: 27099859; PMCID: PMC4832119.

Carter, Katherine, Erin Namovicz, and Deborah M. Weissman. "Domestic Violence and Brain Injury: A Service Provider's Guide." University of North Carolina School of Law, April 2025. https://law.unc.edu/wp-content/uploads/2025/04/DVSP-Brain-Injury-Guide-FINAL.pdf.

Cherian KN, Keynan JN, Anker L, Faerman A, Brown RE, Shamma A, Keynan O, Coetzee JP, Batail JM, Phillips A, Bassano NJ, Sahlem GL, Inzunza J, Millar T, Dickinson J, Rolle CE, Keller J, Adamson M, Kratter IH, Williams NR. Magnesium-ibogaine therapy in veterans with traumatic brain injuries. Nat Med. 2024 Feb;30(2):373-381. doi: 10.1038/s41591-023-02705-w. Epub 2024 Jan 5. PMID: 38182784; PMCID: PMC10878970.

Chun-Pu Chu, Eric, Alan Te-Chang Chen, and Ricky Chiang. "Chiropractic Care of Parkinson's Disease and Deformity." Journal of Life and Medicine 15, no. 5 (May 2022): 717–22. https://doi.org/10.25122/jml-2021-0418.

"Sympathetic Nervous System (SNS): What It Is & Function." Cleveland Clinic, May 21, 2026. https://my.clevelandclinic.org/health/body/23262-sympathetic-nervous-system-sns-fight-or-flight.

Commissioner, Office of the. "Traumatic Brain Injury: What to Know." U.S. Food and Drug Administration. Accessed June 2, 2026. https://www.fda.gov/consumers/consumer-updates/traumatic-brain-injury-what-know-about-symptoms-diagnosis-and-treatment.

Davis, Alan K., Meghan A. DellaCrosse, Nathan D. Sepeda, Adam W. Levin, Mary Cosimano, Hillary Shaub, Taylor Washington, et al. "Five-Year Outcomes of Psilocybin-Assisted

Therapy for Major Depressive Disorder." Journal of Psychedelic Studies 9, no. 4 (November 24, 2025): 320–29. https://doi.org/10.1556/2054.2025.00461.

Dituri, Joseph, and Jason Sonners. The Art and Science of Hyperbaric Medicine. NOW SC Press, 2024.

El Baassiri, Mahmoud G., Zachariah Raouf, Sarah Badin, Alejandro Escobosa, Chhinder P. Sodhi, and Isam W. Nasr. "Dysregulated Brain-Gut Axis in the Setting of Traumatic Brain Injury: Review of Mechanisms and Anti-Inflammatory Pharmacotherapies." Journal of Neuroinflammation 21, no. 1 (May 10, 2024). https://doi.org/10.1186/s12974-024-03118-3.

Espinoza TR, Wright DW. The role of progesterone in traumatic brain injury. The Journal of Head Trauma Rehabilitation. 2011 Nov-Dec;26(6):497-9. doi: 10.1097/HTR.0b013e31823088fa. PMID: 22088981; PMCID: PMC6025750.

Feduccia, Allison A., Lisa Jerome, Berra Yazar-Klosinski, Amy Emerson, Michael C. Mithoefer, and Rick Doblin. "Breakthrough for Trauma Treatment: Safety and Efficacy of MDMA-Assisted Psychotherapy Compared to Paroxetine and Sertraline." Frontiers in Psychiatry 10 (September 12, 2019). https://doi.org/10.3389/fpsyt.2019.00650.

Fitzpatrick Diamond, Patricia F. "Antidepressant Efficacy Called into Question." Genetic Engineering and Biotechnology News, February 1, 2010. https://www.genengnews.com/insights/antidepressant-efficacy-called-into-question/.

Goyal, M, S Singh, E Sibinga, NF Gould, A Rowland-Seymour, R Sharma, Z Berger, et al. "Meditation Programs for

Psychological Stress and Well-Being: A Systematic Review and Meta-Analysis." JAMA Internal Medicine 174, no. 3 (March 2014): 357–68. https://doi.org/10.1016/j.dza.2014.07.007.

Gray SN. An Overview of the Use of Neurofeedback and Biofeedback for the Treatment of Symptoms of Traumatic Brain Injury in Military and Civilian Populations. Medical Acupuncture. 2017 Aug 1;29(4):215-219. doi: 10.1089/acu.2017.1220. PMID: 28874922; PMCID: PMC5580369.

Gukasyan, Natalie, Alan K Davis, Frederick S Barrett, Mary P Cosimano, Nathan D Sepeda, Matthew W Johnson, and Roland R Griffiths. "Efficacy and Safety of Psilocybin-Assisted Treatment for Major Depressive Disorder: Prospective 12-Month Follow-Up." Journal of Psychopharmacology 36, no. 2 (February 2022): 151–58. https://doi.org/10.1177/02698811211073759.

Guo J, Li Z, Yao Y, Fang L, Yu M, Wang Z. Curcumin in the treatment of inflammation and oxidative stress responses in traumatic brain injury: a systematic review and meta-analysis. Front Neurol. 2024 May 10;15:1380353. doi: 10.3389/fneur.2024.1380353. PMID: 38798711; PMCID: PMC11116723.

Hamblin, Michael R. "Photobiomodulation for Traumatic Brain Injury and Stroke." Journal of Neuroscience Research 96, no. 4 (November 13, 2017): 731–43. https://doi.org/10.1002/jnr.24190.

Harej Hrkać A, Pilipović K, Belančić A, Juretić L, Vitezić D, Mršić-Pelčić J. The Therapeutic Potential of Glucagon-like

Peptide 1 Receptor Agonists in Traumatic Brain Injury. Pharmaceuticals (Basel). 2024 Oct 1;17(10):1313. doi: 10.3390/ph17101313. PMID: 39458954; PMCID: PMC11510130.

Hardy, Joseph L, Rolf A. Nelson, Moriah E. Thomason, Daniel A. Sternberg, Kiefer Katovich, Faraz Farzin, and Michael Scanlon. "Enhancing Cognitive Abilities with Comprehensive Training: A Large, Online, Randomized, Active-Controlled Trial." Edited by Mark W. Greenlee. PLoS One 10, no. 9 (September 10, 2015). https://doi.org/10.1371.

Hergert DC, Robertson-Benta C, Sicard V, Schwotzer D, Hutchison K, Covey DP, Quinn DK, Sadek JR, McDonald J, Mayer AR. Use of Medical Cannabis to Treat Traumatic Brain Injury. J Neurotrauma. 2021 Jul 15;38(14):1904-1917. doi: 10.1089/neu.2020.7148. Epub 2021 Jan 25. PMID: 33256496; PMCID: PMC8260892.

Hogenboom, Melissa. "How Ultra-Processed Foods Affect Our Gut Microbiome." BBC, February 20, 2026. https://www.bbc.com/future/article/20260220-how-ultra-processed-foods-influence-our-gut-microbiome.

Institute of Medicine (US) Committee on Nutrition, Trauma and the Brain, Erdman, John, Maria Oria, and Laura Pillsbury, eds. "Nutrition and Traumatic Brain Injury: Improving Acute and Subacute Health Outcomes in Military Personnel ." Institute of Medicine (US) Committee on Nutrition, Trauma, and the Brain, 2011. https://pubmed.ncbi.nlm.nih.gov/24983072/.

Jarosz, Konrad, Klaudyna Kojder, Agata Andrzejewska, Joanna Solek-Pastuszka, and Anna Jurczak. "Cerebrolysin in

Patients with TBI: Systematic Review and Meta-Analysis." Brain Sciences 13, no. 3 (March 17, 2023): 507. https://doi.org/10.3390/brainsci13030506

Jiang, Yuhan, Yili Chen, Youmeng Chen, Xinrong Gong, Zhiyu Chen, and Xin Zhang. "Ketogenic Diet and Gut Microbiota: Exploring New Perspectives on Cognition and Mood." Foods 14, no. 7 (March 30, 2025): 1215. https://doi.org/10.3390/foods14071215.

Khan M, Carter GT, Aggarwal SK, Holland J. Psychedelics for Brain Injury: A Mini-Review. Front Neurol. 2021 Jul 29;12:685085. doi: 10.3389/fneur.2021.685085. Erratum in: Front Neurol. 2021 Sep 30;12:772692. doi: 10.3389/fneur.2021.772692. PMID: 34393973; PMCID: PMC8357986.

Koseli, Eda, Belle Buzzi, Torin Honaker, Yogesh Rakholia, Melissa Lewis, Maya Gaines-Smith, Alaina M. Jaster, Javier Gonzalez-Maeso, and M. Imad Damaj. "Iuphar Article: Psilocybin Induces Long-Lasting Effects via 5-HT2A Receptors in Mouse Models of Chronic Pain." Pharmacological Research 215 (May 2025): 107699. https://doi.org/10.1016/j.phrs.2025.107699.

Krakovski, Maria Alexander, Niraj Arora, Shalini Jain, Jennifer Glover, Keith Dombrowski, Beverly Hernandez, Hariom Yadav, and Anand Karthik Sarma. "Diet-Microbiome-Gut-Brain Nexus in Acute and Chronic Brain Injury." Frontiers in Neuroscience 16 (September 16, 2022). https://doi.org/10.3389/fnins.2022.1002266.

Krygier, Jonathan R., James A.J. Heathers, Sara Shahrestani, Maree Abbott, James J. Gross, and Andrew H. Kemp.

"Mindfulness Meditation, Well-Being, and Heart Rate Variability: A Preliminary Investigation into the Impact of Intensive Vipassana Meditation." International Journal of Psychophysiology 89, no. 3 (September 2013): 305–13. https://doi.org/10.1016/j.ijpsycho.2013.06.017.

Leong, Darryl P, Koon K Teo, Sumathy Rangarajan, Patricio Lopez-Jaramillo, Alvaro Avezum, Andres Orlandini, Pamela Seron, et al. "Prognostic Value of Grip Strength: Findings from the Prospective Urban Rural Epidemiology (PURE) Study." The Lancet 386, no. 9990 (July 18, 2015): 266–73. https://doi.org/10.1016/s0140-6736(14)62000-6.

Lindberg, Megan A., Elisabeth M. Moy Martin, and Donald W. Marion. "Military Traumatic Brain Injury: The History, Impact, and Future." Journal of Neurotrauma 39, no. 17–18 (August 25, 2022): 1133–45. https://doi.org/10.1089/neu.2022.0103.

Lipov E, Sethi Z, Nandra G, Frueh C. Efficacy of combined subanesthetic ketamine infusion and cervical sympathetic blockade as a symptomatic treatment of PTSD/TBI in a special forces patient with a 1-year follow-up: A case report. Heliyon. 2023 Mar 27;9(4):e14891. doi: 10.1016/j.heliyon.2023.e14891. PMID: 37089345; PMCID: PMC10119561.

Liu, Junchang, Gulaisaer Aikebaier, Xusheng Lu, and Xingping Zhang. "Abdominal Massage Modulates Gut Microbiota and Brain-Gut Peptides in Insomnia Model Rats." Frontiers in Microbiology 16 (December 2, 2025). https://doi.org/10.3389/fmicb.2025.1720248.

Loggini A, Tangonan R, El Ammar F, Mansour A, Goldenberg FD, Kramer CL, Lazaridis C. The role of amantadine in cognitive recovery early after traumatic brain injury: A systematic review. Clin Neurol Neurosurg. 2020 Jul;194:105815. doi: 10.1016/j.clineuro.2020.105815. Epub 2020 Mar 21. PMID: 32244036.

Long, Michelle, Justin Lo, and Kaye Pestaina. KFF, March 24, 2026. https://www.kff.org/patient-consumer-protections/claims-denials-and-appeals-in-aca-marketplace-plans-in-2024/.

Longman, Daniel P., Stephen C. Van Hedger, Kirsten McEwan, Eve Griffin, Courtney Hannon, Isabella Harvey, Taisei Kikuta, et al. "Forest Soundscapes Improve Mood, Restoration and Cognition, but Not Physiological Stress or Immunity, Relative to Industrial Soundscapes." Scientific Reports 15, no. 1 (September 30, 2025). https://doi.org/10.1038/s41598-025-11469-x.

Lozano, Diego, Samantha J Schimmel, and Sandra Acosta. "Neuroinflammation in Traumatic Brain Injury: A Chronic Response to an Acute Injury." Brain Circulation 3, no. 3 (2017): 135–42. https://doi.org/10.4103/bc.bc_18_17.

Lucke-Wold BP, Logsdon AF, Nguyen L, Eltanahay A, Turner RC, Bonasso P, Knotts C, Moeck A, Maroon JC, Bailes JE, Rosen CL. Supplements, nutrition, and alternative therapies for the treatment of traumatic brain injury. Nutr Neurosci. 2018 Feb;21(2):79-91. doi: 10.1080/1028415X.2016.1236174. Epub 2016 Oct 5. PMID: 27705610; PMCID: PMC5491366.

Matsuzaki, Rie, Eoin Gunnigle, Violette Geissen, Gerard Clarke, Jatin Nagpal, and John F Cryan. "Pesticide

Exposure and the Microbiota-Gut-Brain Axis." The ISME Journal 17, no. 8 (June 16, 2023): 1153–66. https://doi.org/10.1038/s41396-023-01450-9.

A Multi-Site Phase 3 Study of MDMA-Assisted Therapy for PTSD (MAPP1)." MAPS, December 13, 2023. https://maps.org/mdma/ptsd/mapp1/.

A. Minhas. "Pharma Companies with Active R&D Pipelines Worldwide 2026." Statista, May 11, 2026. https://www.statista.com/statistics/791340/pharmaceutical-companies-number-with-active-pipeline/?srsltid=AfmBOoqnY0zsuhNYIJnqU4HqliXtpFRWyRKTmCn03_4ptOPlg-8FTMLM.

Möhrle, Jörg J. "How Long Does It Take to Develop a New Drug?" The Lancet Regional Health - Europe 43 (July 4, 2024). https://doi.org/10.1016/j.lanepe.2024.100998.

Mooney, James, Mitchell Self, Karim ReFaey, Galal Elsayed, Gustavo Chagoya, Joshua D Bernstock, and James M Johnston. "Concussion in Soccer: A Comprehensive Review of the Literature." Concussion 5, no. 3 (September 2020). https://doi.org/10.2217/cnc-2020-0004.

Mozaffari, Shilan, Roja Rahimi, and Mohammad Abdollahi. "Implications of Melatonin Therapy in Irritable Bowel Syndrome: A Systematic Review." Current Pharmaceutical Design 16, no. 33 (November 1, 2010): 3646–55. https://doi.org/10.2174/138161210794079254.

Mulvaney SW, Lynch JH, Rae Olmsted KL, Mahadevan S, Dineen KJ. The Successful Use of Bilateral 2-Level Ultrasound-Guided Stellate Ganglion Block to Improve Traumatic Brain Injury Symptoms: A

Retrospective Analysis of 23 Patients. Mil Med. 2024 Nov 5;189(11-12):e2573-e2577. doi: 10.1093/milmed/usae193. Erratum for: Mil Med. 2024 Aug 30;189(9-10):253-254. doi: 10.1093/milmed/usae344. PMID: 38771000; PMCID: PMC11536328.

Nedergaard, Jan, Tore Bengtsson, and Barbara Cannon. "Unexpected Evidence for Active Brown Adipose Tissue in Adult Humans." American Journal of Physiology Endocrinology and Metabolism 293, no. 2 (August 2007): 444–52. https://doi.org/10.1152/ajpendo.00691.2006.

Newham, Melissa, and Marica Valente. "The Cost of Influence: How Gifts to Physicians Shape Prescriptions and Drug Costs." Journal of Health Economics 95 (May 2024): 102887. https://doi.org/10.1016/j.jhealeco.2024.102887.

Nguyen BM, Kim D, Bricker S, Bongard F, Neville A, Putnam B, Smith J, Plurad D. Effect of marijuana use on outcomes in traumatic brain injury. Am Surg. 2014 Oct;80(10):979-83. PMID: 25264643.

"How Much Oxygen Comes from the Ocean?" NOAA's National Ocean Service. Accessed June 5, 2026. https://oceanservice.noaa.gov/facts/ocean-oxygen.html.

Nunez, Sergio Gutierrez, Sara Peixoto Rabelo, Nikola Subotic, James Wilson Caruso, and Nebojsa Nick Knezevic. "Chronic Stress and Autoimmunity: The Role of HPA Axis and Cortisol Dysregulation." International Journal of Molecular Sciences 26, no. 20 (October 14, 2025). https://doi.org/10.3390/ijms26209994.

Oschman, James, Gaetan Chevalier, and Richard Brown. "The Effects of Grounding (Earthing) on Inflammation, the

Immune Response, Wound Healing, and Prevention and Treatment of Chronic Inflammatory and Autoimmune Diseases." Journal of Inflammation Research 8 (March 24, 2015): 83–96. https://doi.org/10.2147/jir.s69656.

Pascoe, Michaela C., David R. Thompson, and Chantal F. Ski. "Yoga, Mindfulness-Based Stress Reduction and Stress-Related Physiological Measures: A Meta-Analysis." Psychoneuroendocrinology 86 (December 2017): 152–68. https://doi.org/10.1016/j.psyneuen.2017.08.008.

Peled-Avron, Leehe, Jacob S. Aday, Madeline M. Pantoni, Holly K. Hamilton, and Joshua D. Woolley. "A Meta-Analytic Analysis of the Acute Effects of MDMA on Empathy and Emotion Recognition in Humans." Scientific Reports 15, no. 1 (November 29, 2025). https://doi.org/10.1038/s41598-025-25610-3.

Petrut, Stefana-Maria, Alexandra Maria Bragaru, Alice Elena Munteanu, Adina-Diana Moldovan, Cosmin-Alec Moldovan, and Elena Rusu. "Gut over Mind: Exploring the Powerful Gut–Brain Axis." Nutrients 17, no. 5 (February 28, 2025): 842. https://doi.org/10.3390/nu17050842.

Ririe, Avrina, Nusrat Fatema, Tanni J Dina, Jyothsna Devi Kuchipudi, Prima Tamanna, Libriansyah, Tahmina Akter, and Nafisa Kaderi. "Impact of Microplastic Exposure on Human Health: A Systematic Review of Mechanisms, Biomarkers, and Clinical Outcomes." Cureus, December 28, 2025. https://doi.org/10.7759/cureus.100295.

Sato, Kensuke, Mariko Hara-Chikuma, Masato Yasui, Joe Inoue, and Yun-Gi Kim. "Sufficient Water Intake Maintains the Gut Microbiota and Immune Homeostasis and Promotes

Pathogen Elimination." iScience, May 3, 2024. https://www.cell.com/iscience/fulltext/S2589-0042(24)01125-8.

Sanchez, Gonzalo Moreno, and Alwyn Louise Burridge. "Decision Making in Head Injury Management in the Edwin Smith Papyrus." Neurosurgical Focus 23, no. 1 (July 2007): 1–9. https://doi.org/10.3171/foc-07/07/e5.

Shaito, Abdullah, Hiba Hasan, Karl John Habashy, Walaa Fakih, Samar Abdelhady, Fatima Ahmad, Kazem Zibara, Ali H. Eid, Ahmed F. El-Yazbi, and Firas H. Kobeissy. "Western Diet Aggravates Neuronal Insult in Post-Traumatic Brain Injury: Proposed Pathways for Interplay." EBioMedicine 57 (June 20, 2020): 102829. https://doi.org/10.1016/j.ebiom.2020.102829.

Seligman, Martin E., Tracy A. Steen, Nansook Park, and Christopher Peterson. "Positive Psychology Progress: Empirical Validation of Interventions." American Psychologist 60, no. 5 (2005): 410–21. https://doi.org/10.1037/0003-066x.60.5.410.

Shah, Ruhi K., Justin J. Lin, Tejaswi Makkapati, Arielle A. Berkowitz, and Brian D. Greenwald. "The Effect of Traumatic Brain Injury on the Gastrointestinal System: A Comprehensive Review." Brain Sciences 16, no. 3 (February 25, 2026): 254. https://doi.org/10.3390/brainsci16030254.

Sherrington, Catherine, Anne Tiedemann, Nicola J Fairhall, Sally Hopewell, Zoe A Michaleff, Kirsten Howard, Lindy Clemson, and Sarah E Lamb. "Exercise for Preventing Falls in Older People Living in the Community." Cochrane Database of Systematic Reviews, November 4, 2016. https://doi.org/10.1002/14651858.cd012424.

Sikiric P, Seiwerth S, Rucman R, Kolenc D, Vuletic LB, Drmic D, Grgic T, Strbe S, Zukanovic G, Crvenkovic D, Madzarac G, Rukavina I, Sucic M, Baric M, Starcevic N, Krstonijevic Z, Bencic ML, Filipcic I, Rokotov DS, Vlainic J. Brain-gut Axis and Pentadecapeptide BPC 157: Theoretical and Practical Implications. Curr Neuropharmacol. 2016;14(8):857-865. doi: 10.2174/1570159x1366616050 2153022. PMID: 27138887; PMCID: PMC5333585.

Tang, Yi-Yuan, Britta K. Hölzel, and Michael I. Posner. "The Neuroscience of Mindfulness Meditation." Nature Review Neuroscience 16, no. 4 (March 18, 2015): 213–25. https://doi.org/10.1007/978-3-319-46322-3.

Thakur, Elyse R., Jordan M. Shapiro, Jennifer Wellington, Stephanie J. Sohl, Suzanne C. Danhauer, Baharak Moshiree, Alexander C. Ford, and Kenneth Koch. "A Systematic Review of Yoga for the Treatment of Gastrointestinal Disorders." Neurogastroenterology & Motility 38, no. 1 (September 17, 2024). https://doi.org/10.1111/nmo.14915.

Tournissac, Marine, Philippe Bourassa, Ruben D. Tra-My Vu, Sébastien S. Hébert, Emmanuel Planel, and Frédéric Calon. "Repeated Cold Exposures Protect a Mouse Model of Alzheimer's Disease against Cold-Induced Tau Phosphorylation." Molecular Metabolism 22 (April 2019): 110–20. https://doi.org/10.1016/j.molmet.2019.01.008.

VA Funds First Study on Psychedelic-Assisted Therapy for Veterans." U.S. Department of Veterans Affairs, December 3, 2024. U.S. Department of Veterans Affairs. https://www.va.gov/wilmington-health-care/news-releases/

va-funds-first-study-on-psychedelic-assisted-therapy-for-veterans/.

Wait, Liana. "Study of Former NFL Players Finds 1 in 3 Believes They Have CTE." Harvard Medical School. September 24, 2024. https://hms.harvard.edu/news/study-former-nfl-players-finds-1-3-believes-they-have-cte.

Wei, Yanping, Yifei Xu, Wanlin Chen, Jing Zheng, Hang Chen, and Shulin Chen. "Can Heart Rate Variability Demonstrate the Effects and the Levels of Mindfulness? A Repeated-Measures Study on Experienced and Novice Mindfulness Practitioners." BMC Complementary Medicine and Therapies 25, no. 1 (July 3, 2025). https://doi.org/10.1186/s12906-025-04972-1.

Wielgosz, Joseph, Simon B Goldberg, Tammi R.A. Kral, John D. Dunne, and Richard J. Davidson. "Mindfulness Meditation and Psychopathology." Annual Review of Clinical Psychology 15 (May 2019): 285–316. https://doi.org/10.1146.

Winje, Eirin, Ian Lake, and Simon N. Dankel. "Case Report: Ketogenic Diet Alleviated Anxiety and Depression Associated with Insulin-Dependent Diabetes Management." Frontiers in Nutrition 11 (October 30, 2024). https://doi.org/10.3389/fnut.2024.1404842.

Young, M B, R Andero, K J Ressler, and L.L. Howell. "3,4-Methylenedioxymethamphetamine Facilitates Fear Extinction Learning." Translational Psychiatry 5, no. 9 (September 15, 2015). https://doi.org/10.1038/tp.2015.138.

Yu, Jin, Hong Zhu, Saeid Taheri, William L. Monday, Stephen Perry, and Mark Kindy. "Reduced Neuroinflammation and Improved Functional Recovery after Traumatic Brain Injury by Prophylactic Diet Supplementation in Mice." Nutrients 11, no. 2 (January 31, 2019): 299. https://doi.org/10.3390/nu11020299.

Zanza C, Piccolella F, Racca F, Romenskaya T, Longhitano Y, Franceschi F, Savioli G, Bertozzi G, De Simone S, Cipolloni L, La Russa R. Ketamine in Acute Brain Injury: Current Opinion Following Cerebral Circulation and Electrical Activity. Healthcare (Basel). 2022 Mar 17;10(3):566. doi: 10.3390/healthcare10030566. PMID: 35327044; PMCID: PMC8949520.

Zhao, Xia, Wei Zhang, Ying Zhang, and Xing-An Liu. "Gastrointestinal Dysfunction after Brain Injury: Mechanisms and the Role of the Brain-Gut Axis." World Journal of Gastroenterology 32, no. 10 (March 14, 2026). https://doi.org/10.3748/wjg.v32.i10.115731.

Zou, Bo, Dan Zhao, Shuang Zhou, Jing X. Kang, and Bin Wang. "Insight into the Effects of Omega-3 Fatty Acids on Gut Microbiota: Impact of a Balanced Tissue Omega-6/Omega-3 Ratio." Frontiers in Nutrition 12 (May 16, 2025). https://doi.org/10.3389/fnut.2025.1575323.

www.ingramcontent.com/pod-product-compliance
Lightning Source LLC
LaVergne TN
LVHW090359210926
848480LV00002B/394